S0-BOL-362

—Does your neck, shoulders, or upper back often hurt when you have a headache?

—Are you often tense in your upper body?

—Does your headache cause a viselike pressure around your forehead, scalp, back of head, and/or neck?

—Does your headache pain start when you wake up, start sometime during the day, or interrupt your sleep?

—Do you find it hard to relax?

—Do your headaches start after or during a period of great stress?

If you can relate to these headache descriptions, you may be suffering from a "classic" tension headache—or another of the many types of headache pain that afflict millions of Americans every day. Now you can end that pain with a holistic, noninvasive, multifaceted, completely safe approach to headache relief that takes into account your mind, your body, and your lifestyle. This easy-to-understand, comprehensive guide tells you how!

FREE YOURSELF FROM HEADACHES

DR. JAN STROMFELD is a chiropractor with a private practice located in New York City. He lectures widely on headache prevention and treatment to organizations as diverse as AT&T and the New York City Fire Department. ANITA WEIL is a freelance writer.

FREE YOURSELF FROM HEADACHES

The Natural Drug-Free Program for Prevention and Relief

DR. JAN STROMFELD, D.C.
and
ANITA WEIL

A PLUME BOOK
NEW AMERICAN LIBRARY
A DIVISION OF PENGUIN BOOKS USA INC., NEW YORK
PUBLISHED IN CANADA BY
PENGUIN BOOKS CANADA LIMITED, MARKHAM, ONTARIO

NAL BOOKS ARE AVAILABLE AT QUANTITY DISCOUNTS WHEN USED TO PROMOTE PRODUCTS OR SERVICES. FOR INFORMATION PLEASE WRITE TO PREMIUM MARKETING DIVISION, NEW AMERICAN LIBRARY, 1633 BROADWAY, NEW YORK, NEW YORK 10019.

Copyright © 1989 by Jan Stromfeld and Anita Weil

All rights reserved. For information address New American Library.

Published simultaneously in Canada by Penguin Books Canada Limited.

PLUME TRADEMARK REG. U.S. PAT. OFF. AND FOREIGN COUNTRIES
REGISTERED TRADEMARK—MARCA REGISTRADA
HECHO EN DRESDEN, TN, USA

SIGNET, SIGNET CLASSIC, MENTOR, ONYX, PLUME, MERIDIAN and NAL BOOKS are published *in the United States* by New American Library, a division of Penguin Books USA Inc., 1633 Broadway, New York, New York 10019, *in Canada* by Penguin Books Canada Limited, 2801 John Street, Markham, Ontario L3R 1B4

Library of Congress Cataloging-in-Publication Data

Stromfeld, Jan.
Free yourself from headaches.

1. Headache—Prevention. 2. Headache—Treatment.
I. Weil, Anita. II. Title.
RB128.S84 1989 616.07'2 88-34480
ISBN 0-452-26257-7

First Printing, June, 1989

2 3 4 5 6 7 8 9

PRINTED IN THE UNITED STATES OF AMERICA

Publisher's Note

The ideas, procedures, and suggestions contained in this book are not intended as a substitute for consulting with your physician. All matters regarding your health require medical supervision. The case studies in this book have been fictionalized; however, the conditions and procedures they represent are real.

I would like to dedicate this book to John Upledger, D.O., and John Faye, D.C., for the special roles they have played in my personal and professional lives. Their willingness to share their wealth of knowledge has enabled health professionals around the world to improve the quality of care for millions of patients.

Contents

ACKNOWLEDGMENTS

Our thanks to:

All the scientists, researchers, and health professionals who have helped the health care system evolve into a more natural, comprehensive approach to caring for people.

Special thanks to Pat Warrick for her excellent illustrations.

Faith Hornby Hamlin, our agent, and Alexia Dorszynski, our editor, for their guidance.

Robert Harris for his insight and expert legal advice.

My wife, Ann, for all her love and understanding.

Elaine, Fred, Perry, Ned, and Rory Stromfeld, and Edward and Gussie Berman for the special moments they have shared with me.

Shirley and Gilbert Weil for passing along their love of words and knowledge.

Jonathan Bell for his encouragement and emotional support.

Mary Strudwick for sharing her library, her wisdom, and her generous spirit.

And all the patients who have taken the holistic approach to conquering their headache problems.

INTRODUCTION
A New Approach to Pain Relief

Since you're reading this book, we already know two important things about you: You want to discover how to correct the causes of your headaches, and you're interested in learning how to alleviate pain without drugs.

Free Yourself from Headaches offers you new, holistic answers to the age-old problems of headaches. "Holistic" has its roots in the idea of wholeness: this approach examines the whole person, including structural, chemical, and emotional aspects, in order to discover the underlying causes of maladies. The fundamental concept of holism is that the mind and all parts of the body are connected and interdependent. Therefore, all these components must be considered to create optimal good health. Since headaches occur for a wide variety of reasons, this multifaceted approach is ideal.

Holistic health care incorporates a wide range of modalities, from ancient healing methods to the latest scientific techniques. Since holistic practitioners use only drug-free, noninvasive methods, you don't have to worry about adverse side effects. You will experience positive side effects, however. In addition to helping your headaches, holistic treatment will probably improve many other aspects of your health.

Perhaps you're skeptical because you've been through

the "headache mill" and have tried many doctors and cures without success. If this is the case, we urge you not to give up. Many people have beaten their headache problems through holistic modalities, after conventional methods have failed. You owe it to yourself to consider these new alternatives with an open mind. They have enabled many former headache sufferers to enjoy pain-free lives.

In addition to providing you with easy-to-understand explanations of the causes of headaches and the basis for professional treatments, we offer substantial self-help programs. For example, you will receive step-by-step instructions on a number of relaxation techniques. You will discover how to track down those particular foods and beverages that contribute to your headaches. You will learn self-massage techniques and exercises that can prevent headaches. You will have access to a wide body of information that can substantially enhance your general sense of well-being, as well as eliminate your headaches. This information is summarized and organized for easy application in the Holistic Headache Recovery Program (see pp. 194–205).

The holistic approach may be new to you, but it has already gained a great number of adherents. As people become increasingly educated about their health, the popularity of the holistic health care system is growing. Millions are learning to banish nagging health problems such as headaches. They are helping themselves and also seeking out holistically oriented health professionals with a wide range of specialties. Encouraging this trend are many enlightened medical doctors, who recommend alternative methods in appropriate cases. Trying the holistic approach need not mean giving up your trusted family doctor or totally changing your orientation. It means expanding your options and exploring new options.

There is a new age of health care dawning. We invite you to share in its benefits. The holistic path may lead you to a healthier, happier, headache-free life.

Chapter One

The Holistic Approach

SINCE PREHISTORIC TIMES, PEOPLE HAVE BEEN SEARCHING for headache cures. Archeologists have discovered skulls from the Neolithic and Bronze ages with holes drilled in them. This may have been a desperate attempt to free headache sufferers from the "demons" causing their problems. Many ancient cultures believed that the gods inflicted headaches upon mankind as punishment.

During Greece's golden age, such natural cures as willow bark, mandrake root, sarsaparilla, and tiger balm were used to relieve headache pain. In medieval times, treatments regressed into the realm of the bizarre, and reptiles' skin, beavers' testicles, cows' brains, powdered flies, live toads, dead buzzards, and leeches were applied to the skin of headache victims. Hot irons were sometimes placed directly on the forehead. In some cases, an incision was made in the head and garlic or dill was placed directly inside. One medical doctrine of these dark ages recommended using walnuts to cure headaches because walnuts resemble the cerebral cortex in appearance.

We've come a long way since those days. Modern remedies are not nearly so horrific. They are not totally safe, however. The drugs that are so commonly used to combat headaches can have dangerous side effects, especially if they are used too often.

The Dangers of Standard Drug Treatment

Each year, Americans consume an estimated fifty million pounds of *aspirin*. Some headache sufferers routinely take as many as ten tablets a day. While aspirin can be a wonderfully helpful drug, doses this large can take their toll. Aspirin can upset the gastrointestinal system by irritating the mucous membranes in the digestive tract, causing stomach cramps, nausea, heartburn, and blood in the stool. Lowered red blood cell production and a reduced ability of the blood to clot have also been reported.

One of the greatest dangers of aspirin and most other drugs is the rebound effect. After the drug wears off, pain may intensify, creating both the need for more medication for relief and psychological dependency. Agitation, cramps, and increased head pain may ensue when the drug is discontinued.

Acetaminophen, commonly found in Tylenol and other over-the-counter pain medications, has been touted as a safer alternative to aspirin. Although it is true that acetaminophen does not cause the same adverse gastrointestinal effects, overuse can cause abnormalities in the liver and kidneys—and it's easier to overdose on acetaminophen than on aspirin. *Ibuprofen*, an anti-inflammatory drug, is now being recommended. Some of its possible side effects include gastrointestinal bleeding or perforation and changes in vision.

Sinus headache remedies and other over-the-counter combinations often contain *caffeine*, which can cause symptoms such as sleep disturbances, heart palpitations, digestive disorders, hypertension, and emotional distress. Sinus combinations often include decongestants, which, if overused, can increase blood pressure and affect circulation.

Tranquilizers are sometimes prescribed to headache patients to reduce tension. Loss of coordination, drowsiness, weight gain, depression, dependence, and addiction are among the pitfalls of prolonged use of tranquilizers. *Antidepressants* are sometimes prescribed to combat the depression that can arise from enduring chronic head pain. Some of the potential side effects of antidepressants include constipation, weight gain, blurred vision, and cardiovascular problems.

Migraine patients are often given *ergotamine tartrate*, a blood vessel dilator; overdosage can cause hallucinations, seizures, and blood vessel constriction. Other potential side effects include cramps, numbness, tingling and swelling in the extremities, chest pain, and changes in the heart rate. *Methysergide*, a drug that must be taken on a daily basis to prevent migraines and cluster headaches, can cause the development of scar tissue on the organs and impair blood circulation. Stomach pains, sleeplessness, and hallucinations can also result. *Propanol hydrochloride* is another daily migraine/cluster medication. It can cause weight gain, fatigue, stomach upset, and affect the blood pressure and heart. It is especially dangerous for pregnant women.

This information is not meant to terrify or depress you. It is meant to alert you to the possible hazards of drugs you might be taking and make you aware that it is usually best to use natural headache cures. Although many patients can take medication without any adverse side effects, new side effects of drugs that were once considered harmless are often discovered years later. Doesn't it make more sense to correct the causes of your headaches than merely to treat the symptoms with drugs?

The idea of giving up medications—even aspirin—may seem intimidating or frightening to you now. But once you discover the breadth and versatility of the holistic approach, you will no longer have reason to be afraid. Let's look at two case histories of people who learned to control their headaches without drugs.

Holistic Case Histories

Jennifer R. was working on her computer when a glaring zigzag pattern suddenly obliterated half of her vision. She felt a wave of nausea, mixed with panic and dread. Half-blinded by the pulsing pattern, she stumbled to the office bathroom. Crouching in the corner, she waited for the hallucinations to subside. What followed was worse: deep throbbing pain that spread from one side of her face to the other. The pain was so intense that she couldn't work the rest of the day, nor could she drive home. Moaning in agony, she spent the rest of the afternoon curled up on the bathroom floor.

Like an estimated fifteen million other Americans, Jennifer suffered from migraine attacks at least once a month. "Sometimes the pain was so bad, I almost wanted to cut my head off," she said. Over the years, she had gone to several doctors. They had prescribed drugs that produced distressing side effects such as nausea, vomiting, dizziness, and extreme drowsiness.

Drugs were not the answer to Jennifer's problem; in fact, they were a primary cause. When Jennifer went to a holistically oriented doctor, he suggested that she stop taking birth control pills. Once she did, the frequency of her migraine attacks was immediately reduced. Since her doctor also suspected that diet was a factor in her case, he encouraged Jennifer to go on a special diet that eliminated substances that often trigger migraines. After a few months of this program, she stopped having migraines altogether.

"I felt like I was released from prison," said Jennifer. "For the first time in years, I would wake up in the morning without worrying that I'd have an attack that day. What an incredible relief!"

Matt S. was one of approximately twenty-five million Americans who endure frequent tension headaches due to muscle contraction. "I couldn't understand it," said Matt. "It was especially frustrating because I prided myself on having a healthy lifestyle." Matt gulped megavitamins, bought lunch at the salad bar, worked out at the health club, and stayed away from drugs, alcohol, and caffeine. "I didn't like taking painkillers, but I didn't know what else to do. The headaches were really making my life miserable."

When we examined Matt, we discovered that he was undermining his healthy lifestyle with one bad habit: He spent hours at work holding the telephone between his ear and shoulder. This had caused biomechanical problems in his neck leading to restricted movement of his cervical (neck) vertebrae (spinal bones). The outcome of this was irritation to his nervous system as well as to the blood vessels supplying his head, resulting in headaches.

Gentle chiropractic manipulation served to realign his vertebrae and free the impinged nerves and blood vessels. As a preventive measure, Matt bought a set of headphones to use at work. Whenever he felt tension gathering in his neck, he took a little "stretching break" to carefully stretch and massage his neck. Headaches were no longer a part of his life.

You, too, can benefit from the holistic approach, whether you suffer from tension headaches, migraine or cluster headaches, pain related to sinus problems, TMJ (temporomandibular joint) syndrome, hypoglycemia, allergies, or more obscure conditions. You need no longer feel like a helpless victim. You can take control over your health and your life.

The History of Holism

You may be wary of the holistic approach because you suspect it is "trendy," new, or unproven. In fact, although holism has become more widely developed and accepted in the last two decades, it has ancient roots.

Thousands of years ago, Chinese doctors developed a system for balancing the energy currents in the body. This system must have been quite successful: The doctors were paid to keep their patients well and, if the patient became ill, payment was withheld. Aspects of the Chinese medical system, such as acupuncture and shiatsu massage, are still widely used and have gained the respect of Westerners.

Another ancient holistic health care system that is still widely employed is Ayurvedic. This Indian system utilizes personalized programs of dietary changes, meditation, and yoga to restore balance to the body. Yoga has been a popular way to keep both the mind and the body fit for over a thousand years.

Hippocrates, the father of medicine, might also be called the father of chiropractic, since he made the connection between spinal misalignments and sickness and performed spinal adjustments. His writings showed that he was aware of the body's ability to heal itself, an important component of holism.

Until the mid-seventeenth century, most learned people considered the mind, body, and spirit to be one interconnected entity. Then the philosopher Descartes introduced the idea of the duality of the mind and body, and Cartesian philosophy gained prominence in Europe. In the East, however, health practitioners still worked with modalities that respected the connection between the mind and the body.

During the last three centuries in Europe and its colonies, the upper classes generally came under the care of medical doctors, but the masses relied on herbalists, midwives, botanic doctors, and bonesetters. These natural healers won the trust and gratitude of many patients. In the early part of the twentieth century, chiropractic and homeopathy gained a great number of adherents.

In the 1960s many seekers discovered the benefits of yoga, massage, herbs, and the ability of the mind to heal the body. The 1970s saw a fitness explosion as scores of people took up jogging, aerobic dance, or other forms of exercise and changed their diets to reduce calories and cholesterol. At the same time, many people became involved in human potential movements or began practicing Transcendental Meditation and other forms of the ancient art of meditation.

While some of this exploration was superficial and transient, it brought fundamental and lasting change to the lives of a great number of people. They sought to become more actively involved in maintaining their health and to steer clear of medication and surgery whenever possible. Alternative health care began to flourish and expand.

There are now many holistic health care centers throughout the world. Holistic medical doctors, holistic chiropractors, physical therapists, massage therapists, and many other holistically oriented specialists treat millions of patients. The health care system is in the process of evolving into taking a more naturally oriented approach for correcting bodily ailments.

The Components of Holistic Health Care

The word "holistic" comes from the word "whole." The holistic health care system treats *all* aspects of the *whole* person. In holistic care, the complex interaction of the structural, chemical, and emotional components of the individual are evaluated and balanced.

The structural component of your body involves your fascia (connective tissue), muscles, ligaments, tendons, and bones. This musculoskeletal structure is the foundation of your body. Just as buildings need a strong and balanced foundation, so do human beings. If there are imbalances or weaknesses in your structure, health problems, such as headaches, can develop. The holistic professional can make adjustments to correct structural imbalances. He or she can also educate you as to how you can maintain balance in your body and strengthen your structure through healthy habits.

The chemical component concerns your hormonal, circulatory, and digestive systems and their interaction. Taking into consideration the unique chemistry of your body, this aspect of holistic health care involves the role of nutrition, vitamins, minerals, and food allergies.

The emotional aspect of the holistic approach considers your personality, lifestyle, and psychological and spiritual condition. Emotions can have a profound effect on health; specifically, headaches can result from unresolved tension and emotional conflicts. It's not that we believe headaches are "all in your head," but rather that we understand that the mind and the body directly affect each other. Dealing with stress and emotional issues in a positive way can have a remarkable effect on your health and headaches.

The Holistic Modalities

The holistic health care system encompasses such a large number of modalities that it would be difficult to cover them all in one volume. We have carefully selected those methods that we have found to be most successful in treating headaches:

- Chiropractic. This is the largest alternative health care system in the country, treating millions of Americans each year. Doctors of chiropractic (also known as chiropractors or chiropractic physicians) use a wide range of natural therapies to correct physical ailments. They work to create optimal well-being by giving special attention to spinal biomechanics, the nervous system, the musculolskeletal system, and nutritional and environmental factors.
- Craniosacral Therapy. This approach is designed to restore normal functioning to the cranium (skull) and the nervous, musculoskeletal, and other systems of the body. Gentle manipulation of the bony structures and soft tissues is employed.
- Nutritional Counseling. Good nutrition is a prerequisite for good health. In a later chapter, we will explore the fundamentals of healthy eating and vitamin/mineral/herbal supplementation. Since food allergies are a common cause of headaches, you will be given a method for detecting those foods you are allergic to and must avoid. We will also discuss blood sugar imbalances that can lead to headaches and substances that frequently trigger migraine headaches.
- Psychological Techniques. Psychological stress contributes not only to tension headaches, but also to most other types. We will teach you how

to reduce stress by presenting a number of easy-to-use techniques. We will also explore means of coping with the psychological and emotional aspects of headaches.

- Yoga and Therapeutic Exercise. Many modern forms of therapeutic exercise are based on yoga, one of the oldest and wisest self-care systems. We will present exercises that can help prevent headaches. We will also discuss how to modify your daily habits to reduce the stress on your body that can lead to headaches.
- Massage. There are many forms of this ancient healing art. We will focus on classical massage, finger pressure therapy, reflexology, and hot compress therapy for headache relief and prevention. We will also teach you self-massage techniques to prevent and alleviate pain.

The Patient As a Partner

Headaches are a signal that something is wrong. If you smother that signal with drugs, the root causes will remain uncorrected and the headaches will most likely recur. Instead of merely treating the symptoms with drugs, holistic practitioners try to discover what your body is trying to tell you. Once that is determined, steps are taken to give your body what it needs, whether that is professional treatment or a simple change in habits. Then the innate self-correcting mechanisms of your body can take over and maintain homeostasis—normal, healthy functioning.

Education is an important part of holistic health care. Practitioners educate their patients on maintaining good health and preventing pain from recurring once balance has been restored. You do not need a Ph.D.; a basic comprehension of how your body works is sufficient. You will be pleasantly surprised to see how easy it is to learn the basics of healthy living—and that knowledge will give you greater control over your body and headaches. Headaches will not seem as terrifying and overwhelming once you understand them.

Holistically oriented health professionals are aware of the importance of combining modern scientific approaches with old-fashioned values. A loving touch and a caring attitude are as important as professional competence.

The holistic professional can be an architect who creates the blueprint for your health. However, you must become a partner in building and maintaining a strong, healthy body. Your body is your home, and, like any home, it needs care if it is to be a comfortable place. While much can be done for you, *you* are the one who is ultimately in control.

This responsibility may sound awesome at first, but when you consider it thoughtfully, it makes perfect sense. After all, who cares more about your body than you do? Who knows how your body feels better than you do?

Taking responsibility for your own health does not mean doing everything on your own. You should still turn to professionals for guidance, correction, and help. But it is up to you to take the preventive measures that are so important in conquering headaches.

Prevention

"Prevention is better than cure," says the ancient proverb, and it remains true today. Isn't it more sensible to treat yourself well and avoid headaches than to hope for a miracle cure? Prevention is an integral part of the holistic approach. When healthy living becomes a way of life, headaches are much less likely to strike.

Prevention of headaches has many facets: posture, work and personal habits, food and drink intake, relaxation and stretching. We will give you step-by-step advice concerning all these matters, and much more. You needn't worry that you have to become a "health nut" or sacrifice everything you enjoy; you may need to modify a few habits, but you are likely to enjoy the changes. And you will be gaining far more than you will be giving up.

A Word of Warning

Although most headaches are the result of minor problems in lifestyle, headaches *can* be symptoms of serious organic illnesses. They may indicate a brain tumor, brain hemorrhaging, meningitis, temporal arteritis, glaucoma, infection, head trauma, or other diseases.

The headaches that are symptomatic of major diseases are not always distinct from ordinary headaches; therefore, self-diagnosis is not sufficient. Medical tests are necessary to rule out the possibility of life-threatening illnesses. The majority of people who have headaches are not suffering from serious disease; there is no need to panic, but it's wise to play it safe. We strongly recommend that you undergo a complete medical examination before beginning the Holistic Headache Recovery Program.

Once your physician rules out the presence of any disease, you will be ready to begin the process of discovering why you have headaches and how to go about correcting these causes through natural methods. You will be ready to embark on the holistic path. All it takes is an honest commitment to do what you can to free yourself from pain.

Chapter Two

Health Begins with Understanding

HEADACHES CAUSE PAIN. BUT WHAT EXACTLY IS PAIN? LET'S take a detailed look at our bodies to discover the mechanics of pain, how it is created and interpreted.

Our bodies are controlled by two systems: the nervous system and the endocrine, or hormonal, system. The feeling or sensation of pain is created within the nervous system, which consists of the brain, spinal cord, and the nerves that run throughout the entire body. The nervous system forms a complex communication network within the body, enabling all parts to communicate with the brain and vice versa.

Nerves are made up of small components called nerve cells. Each cell has two ends: the receiver end, or dendrite, which receives messages, and the transmitter end, or axon, which transmits messages and signals to the next nerve cell. Pain signals travel from the transmitter end of one cell to the receiver end of the next cell across a junction between the cells called a synapse.

The transmission of the pain message at the synapse is influenced by neurotransmitters—chemicals that are activated by pain signals. Some of the neurotransmitters involved are called serotonin, dopamine, norepinephrine, and acetylcholine. Many medications are designed to block pain messages at the synapse.

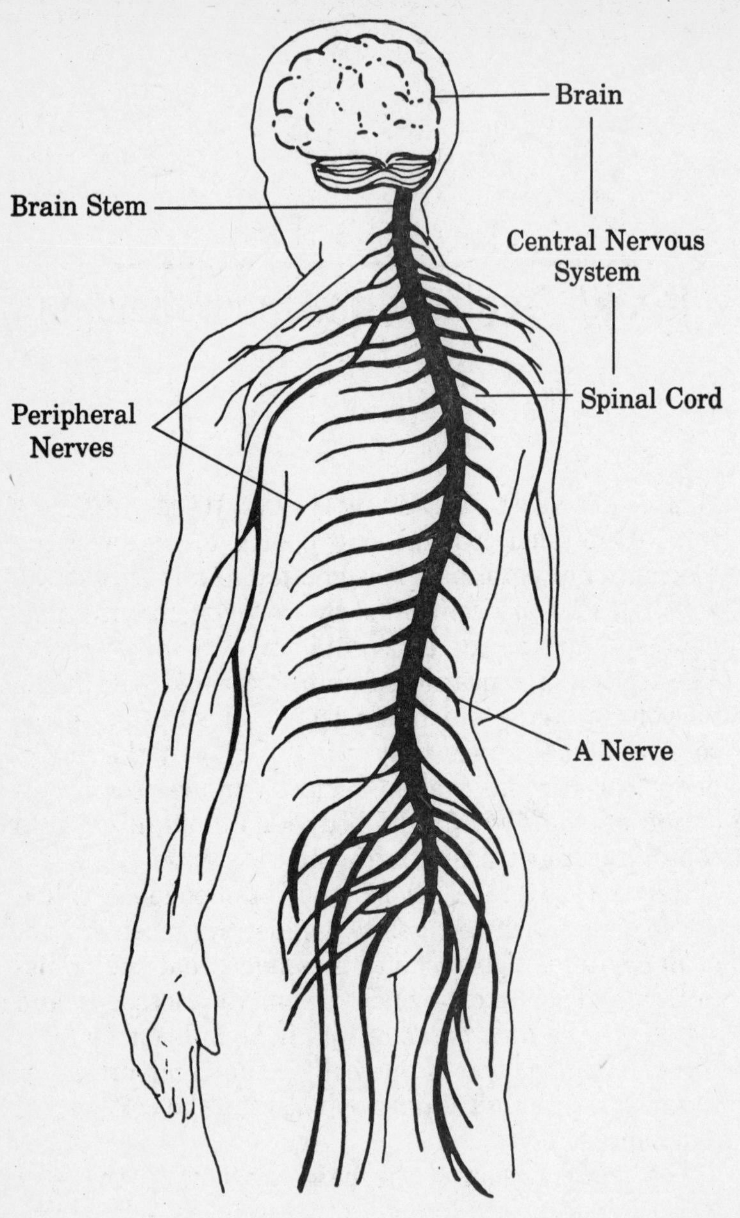

The Nervous System

If the pain message is not blocked at the synapse, it travels through the nerves into the spinal cord, then up the spinal cord into the brain.

The pain signals associated with headaches usually originate from one of six main causes:

- Overcontraction or tightening of the muscles of the head, scalp, face, jaw, or neck.
- Alterations in the fluid pressure within the skull.
- Changes in the blood vessels of the head, scalp, face, jaw, or neck.
- Chemical changes, such as blood sugar fluctuations, hormonal shifts, or allergic responses, especially those due to food allergy reactions.
- Spinal problems, pinched nerves, or other adverse changes affecting the functioning of the nervous system.
- Restrictions in the movements of the cranial bones that make up the skull, including the temporomandibular joint (TMJ), or jaw.

Our goal is to eliminate your fear and confusion regarding headaches and to help you discover the causes of your headaches and how to eliminate them.

Common Causes of Chronic Pain

Let's examine some of the common, yet frequently overlooked, causes of chronic pain and headaches.

Pinched Nerves

The spine (backbone) is composed of vertebral bones separated by cushions called discs. The spine is designed to go through certain ranges of motion, but often parts of the spine develop restrictions and are unable to move properly. This is called hypomobility. It leads to altered biomechanics and frequently causes a pinching or irritation to the nerves passing between the bones. Pinched nerves can lead to a host of health problems, including frequent headaches. Many people with pinched nerves don't even realize that they have them, but they often develop chronic pain as a result.

Restricted Blood Flow

The vertebral arteries, which supply blood to the head, pass through the cervical (neck) region of the spine. If the spine is out of balance and is twisted in the neck region, interference with the normal blood flow to the brain can result, causing headaches.

Cranial Imbalances

The skull (cranium) is composed of small bones, many of which overlap each other. The cranial bones are designed to make small movements to help pump fluid around the brain and down the spinal cord. Often these cranial bones become jammed or stuck to each other. This can cause changes in the blood vessels and fluid pressure in the skull, as well as changes in the muscles and membranes of the scalp, head, and neck. The end result can be chronic headaches as well as neck pain and other problems.

Modern chiropractors are trained in locating, evaluating, and correcting nerve and muscle problems. Therefore, we believe that a chiropractic examination is an integral component of the holistic approach to dealing with chronic headaches.

The Gate Control Theory

The Gate Control theory of pain was developed in the mid-sixties by Drs. Ronald Melzack and Patrick Wall. They postulated that a specialized group of nerve cells in the spinal cord function as a "gate" to regulate transmission of pain signals. According to their theory, large bundles of nerve fibers, which signal the sensation of touch, can close the gate, thus stopping transmission to the brain, while smaller bundles of fibers, which signal the sensation of pain, can keep it open. This led to the idea that overloading the larger "touch" fibers, whose signals travel faster, might close off the gate to the pain fibers, thereby interfering with the feeling of pain. This may account for the natural instinct to rub one's forehead during a headache. Rubbing stimulates the touch fibers, which may close off the gate to the pain fibers.

A pain relief technique called TENS (transcutaneous electrical nerve stimulation) evolved out of the Gate Control theory. TENS involves placing electrodes on the skin above the source of the pain. These are attached to an electrical unit, which sends a calibrated pulsation through the electrodes. The purpose is to overload the larger touch fibers, thereby closing the gate to pain signals. In some cases, this has been found to reduce the experience of pain.

The Biochemistry of Pain

Neurokinins are protein substances found in our bodies; they are thought to intensify pain. Some researchers believe that experiencing pain or injury causes the neurokinins to break out of storage and flood the system. Neurokinins may also be released during migraines, thereby lowering the pain threshold and increasing the experience of pain associated with these headaches.

Serotonins are neurotransmitters synthesized within our bodies from the amino acid L-tryptophan. They are believed to regulate the body's response to stress and produce feelings of relaxation. Some people find it helpful to take the amino acid L-tryptophan in supplement form, along with B-vitamins, to increase the production of serotonins. L-tryptophan is also found naturally in green leafy vegetables, dairy products, and some fruits.

The Placebo Response

A placebo is a treatment that has no concrete physiological value. The most common form of placebos are sugar pills with no active ingredients. Yet studies have shown that approximately 40 percent of a group of people suffering from headaches will report feeling relief after receiving the placebo. This has been proven time and time again, since placebos are constantly used in testing new medications.

What is to account for this amazing phenomenon? Many researchers believe that placebos involve a form of self-hypnosis, during which the patients convince themselves that they will feel better. The beneficial effect may also reflect faith in the person who dispenses the placebo. The impact of faith is dramatically demonstrated by religious leaders who practice faith healing. In many cases, the recoveries they elicit are genuine; but whether they are acts of God or the result of the faith in the power of God to heal depends on personal beliefs. Whatever the precise mechanism of the placebo response, it certainly proves that faith in the treatment and in the possibility of success play a vital role in recovery.

There are many ways to unleash the power of your mind to control pain. Neurolinguistic programming (NLP), creative visualization, relaxation, and meditation are some of the techniques you will learn about in this book. These techniques can help activate your body's natural healing response and counteract the effects of stress. They also help stimulate the production of endorphins, nature's painkillers.

Endorphins

The body produces its own painkillers, which have a structure very similar to morphine. These natural painkillers, called endorphins, alter nerve transmission in a manner that lessens pain. Endorphins may be responsible for previously unexplained phenomenon, such as wounded soldiers who feel no pain until they leave the battlefield or athletes who do not feel an injury until the game ends. Stepped-up endorphin production may be responsible for the ability of some people to walk on fire or lie on a bed of nails without feeling pain.

Exercise can raise the endorphin level, which may account for the feeling of "runner's high." There may be some scientific basis behind the saying, "Laughter is the best medicine," since laughter stimulates endorphin production. So does being in love. Bringing more love and laughter into your life may help your headache problem, and it certainly can't hurt.

Personal Aspects of Pain

You now know something about the physiological mechanisms behind head pain. But pain is much more than nerve impulses and chemical reactions. Emotions, expectations, fears, beliefs, and other psychological factors are highly involved in your experience of pain. So is your personality.

The following quiz is designed to start you thinking about the psychological aspects of headaches. It will help you become aware of any subconscious beliefs you may hold regarding headaches. Often, the simple act of acknowledging your greatest fears on a conscious level can take away their frightening power. This is, of course, the basis behind most forms of psychotherapy.

Ask yourself the following questions:

- When did you first start getting headaches? What was going on emotionally in your life at that time?
- Do you believe it is inevitable that you will suffer from headaches because your parents did?
- Do you think headaches are a punishment or a form of divine retribution for something you have done in the past?
- Do you feel you deserve headaches for any reason?
- Do you think the headaches are your fault because they result from stress?
- Do you feel headaches are a sign of weakness or character deficiency?
- Do you use headaches as an excuse to avoid doing things you don't want to do?
- Are your headaches a cry for help, love, nurturing, and/or attention?
- Do you think of your body as being a hostile, separate entity from your mind and soul?
- Do you think headaches strike at random and that you have no control over them?
- Do you enjoy life? Do you look forward to your days or dread them?

- Are you a perfectionist? Are you harsh, judgmental, or overdemanding with yourself?
- Do you love yourself? Do you love others?
- Do you experience a great deal of anger toward yourself? Toward others?
- Are you frequently afraid, anxious, frustrated, or depressed?

Some of your responses to these questions may, initially, be disturbing. But it is better to acknowledge them than to let them fester in your unconscious. Remember that you are not alone; many other people experience the same doubts and fears. Don't blame yourself if some of these responses seem illogical. Your feelings are always valid; don't try to deny them even if they are unpleasant. Accept them. Accept yourself for who you are right here and now. Then read on and learn how to let go of the negative thoughts that might be contributing to your pain problem.

Inheriting Pain

Josephine R., a divorced woman in her mid-thirties, endured tension headaches about four times a week. She frequently complained about her pain to anyone who would listen, which made her quite unpopular. Food provided consolation, and she put on a lot of weight; she also relied on Valium and Percodan to cope with her pain and unhappiness.

"My father had headaches all his life. I thought I had inherited them from him. I thought I was genetically doomed," said Josephine.

An article on drug-free headache relief spurred her to visit a holistic doctor. A multifaceted examination yielded evidence of food allergies and structural problems in the TMJ. Both of these problems stemmed from her unhappy childhood and her unresolved anger toward her father.

The suppressed rage caused Josephine to tighten the muscles of her jaw during sleep, which created problems in the TMJ. Her unhappy experiences with her father also led her to distrust men in general, which made it difficult for her to have a fulfilling relationship. To fill the void created by a lack of love in her life, she overindulged in many of the wrong foods, developing food allergies. Therefore, although she had not inherited headaches from her father directly, she had done so indirectly. Her father had left her burdened with a psychological legacy that caused her to develop physical problems and headaches.

Josephine's doctor used a special procedure called somato emotional release, which will be explained in detail in a later chapter (p. 122). Through this method, Josephine was able to let go of much of her anger. After the underlying emotional conflict was released, her doctor took steps to correct her food allergy reactions and her TMJ problems. Josephine's headaches diminished and her personal life took on a whole new positive direction.

Like Josephine's doctor, we encourage you to abandon the view that you are fated to endure a lifetime of headaches if your parents did. Instead, devote your energy to discovering how you can correct other factors that are causing your headaches. Even if there is a genetic factor, you can learn about ways to help your headaches and can avoid suffering as your parents did.

Learning to Hurt

Although the question of genetic inheritance of headaches is debatable, we do know that response to pain is shaped during the early childhood years. In a sense, pain is a learned phenomenon. Studies have shown that the way our parents and other figures of authority reacted to our earliest injuries and sicknesses has a direct effect on how we experience pain as adults.

If our parents responded to our hurts with excessive love, attention, and sympathy, we may develop a low pain threshold and feel pain easily and intensely. We may unconsciously manifest headaches as a way of gaining attention. Headaches may be a way to manipulate people into giving us what we feel we cannot get in other ways.

If our parents overresponded to our pain, this can create a sense of the world being an unsafe place. We may grow up to be anxious and nervous, which can result in experiencing more of the very pain that we fear. If our parents encouraged us to make a quick recovery and did not place too much emphasis on the pain, we are less likely to be fearful and anxious as adults. If our parents responded effectively to our pain during the formative years, we may have developed a high pain threshold and not feel pain easily.

In addition to parental response, pain perception is also affected by the birth experience, by age, and by gender. Many men have a tendency to think of pain, both emotional and physical, as a sign of weakness. This is one reason why many more women than men buy self-help books, and why women also visit health professionals more readily.

Don't let yourself be trapped into thinking that pain is a sign of weakness or a lack of strength. Pain is part of being human. Admitting that you have a headache problem shouldn't be interpreted as a character flaw and lower your self-esteem. In fact, actively seeking help is a sign of healthy self-esteem and self-respect.

Pain Is Not Punishment

Nina M. became pregnant when she was sixteen. Marriage was out of the question, and she was ashamed to tell her parents, who were deeply religious. Although she felt tremendously guilty, she underwent an abortion on her own. Soon afterward, she began suffering from terrible headaches, often so severe that she had to leave school in the middle of a class. Her grades suffered, and so did her social life.

"I was sure the headaches were a punishment from God," Nina said. "I didn't even bother to try to get help because I thought I deserved to suffer."

After taking a psychology course in college, Nina decided to find a counselor. The therapist was the first person she had ever told about the abortion, and she felt a great deal of relief when she unburdened herself. This alone did not clear up her headaches. However, the therapy did help her realize that she did not deserve to suffer, and so she actively sought and found relief.

The word "pain" comes from the Latin word *poena,* meaning punishment. Many ancient peoples believed that pain was a punishment from the gods. Even today, many dictionaries include "punishment or penalty" as one of the definitions of pain. And many people feel, if only on a subconscious level, that head pain is a punishment for something they did wrong. "What did I do to deserve this?" is a common lament.

Perhaps you have done something wrong in your life; most people have. There is no reason to believe that headaches are a form of punishment, however. First of all, it's unlikely that your wrongdoing would warrant such a cruel penalty. Second, headaches strike even the most well-behaved people. Headaches cross all barriers, striking saints and sinners alike. You should not believe you have been singled out for divine retribution; this belief can cause more headaches to occur and thwart your chances for recovery. Instead of devoting energy to negative beliefs, you can learn to use the power of your mind to create good health.

You Are Not to Blame

The friends and families of headache sufferers sometimes exhibit a lack of sympathy and patience because they believe the pain is "all in your head." "If you could just relax and not get so uptight, you wouldn't get headaches," they might say. Since it is well known that headaches can have an emotional component, some people believe that the pain is not "real" and not as deserving of compassion as other ailments. If you suffer from headaches, you know that the pain is, indeed, very real. There may well be contributing emotional factors, but these can cause substantial structural and chemical disturbances. In the holistic health professions we are more concerned with understanding the interaction of the mind and body than with labeling certain ailments physical and others psychosomatic.

Emotional, chemical, and structural threads all weave into the cloth of health. If one strand is pulled, the others may unravel. Instead of trying to separate these threads, we holistic practitioners strive to connect them. We work to balance the mind and the body.

It is important that you relieve yourself of the burden of blame. Everyone has troubling feelings, but people vent them in different ways. For example, job tension might result in an angry outburst at a colleague, in the desire for a couple of cocktails, or in a throbbing headache. Yes, stress and other emotional factors may be involved in your headache problem. But this does not mean the headaches are "your fault."

Are You Trying to Avoid Something?

"Not tonight dear, I have a headache," is an old and famous excuse for avoiding sex. Although few people actually use headaches to avoid sex, many use them to avoid other things. Chronic pain may provide a convenient excuse for not making changes in your life, such as taking on a more challenging job or getting involved in a new relationship. Headaches can also be a way of trying to avoid responsibilities when they seem overwhelming. This usually takes place on a subconscious level and should not be a cause for shame or guilt.

Eddie B.'s headaches began when he was eight years old. He had just moved to a new neighborhood and as a result was the class scapegoat. Headaches gave him a chance to stay home with his loving mother instead of facing his taunting classmates. The headaches were genuine; so was the desire to avoid going to school.

Unfortunately, habits often outlive their usefulness. Eddie's chronic headaches continued into his adulthood. But once he was working, he couldn't afford to stay home in bed and read comic books. He started taking pills to ease the pain. But the pills made him so drowsy that he couldn't concentrate, and his work deteriorated. Fortunately, Eddie had a loving wife who was concerned about his growing dependence on painkillers. She urged him to learn relaxation methods to reduce his tension level. She also encouraged him not to drive himself so hard at work, not to be a perfectionist, not to take on so many overtime assignments. Once Eddie allowed himself the breaks he needed for healthy functioning, his headaches became infrequent occurrences instead of a constant torment.

Ask yourself honestly if you use headaches as a means of avoidance. If this is a possibility, what you need to do is take action to change whatever it is you find unpleasant and want to avoid. Would you like a different job? Do you yearn to move to a different environment? Do you need to have a little more private time away from your children? Should you work on your love relationship in order to make it more satisfying?

It is not easy to make these fundamental changes in your life, but neither is it easy to endure chronic headaches. And making changes may cost money, but so do doctors' appointments and medication. In the long run, adapting your lifestyle may be the least painful solution.

Pain Is a Message

Headaches are a message that something is wrong. They may be trying to tell you a myriad of things. You may have chemical or structural imbalances that need to be diagnosed and corrected. Perhaps you need to change your lifestyle to reduce frustration and anxiety. It may help to release built-up anger. You may need more love or attention. Perhaps you should be easier on yourself and/or on others. Or maybe you simply need to slow down.

It could be that headaches are a message that you should practice relaxation techniques or new forms of exercise; that your posture or work habits are unhealthy; that you need spinal adjustments; that changes should be made in your diet; that you need more or less sleep; that you are taking some medication that is doing you harm, or that you need vitamin and mineral supplementation. These are only some of the messages your headaches may be trying to get across.

Headaches can, in fact, be helpful. They can be your body's way of trying to prevent more damage from being done.

Reading the Signals: The Headache Diary

An effective way to read the signals is to keep a headache diary. The purpose of the diary is to help you recognize contributing factors and make necessary changes.

Use one piece of paper for each week. Divide it into the days of the week. In each day's section, write down what your major activities were and how you felt emotionally. Also jot down any events or interactions that affected your emotional state. If you had a headache that day, print a large *H* in that section and note the duration and intensity of the pain.

You might make your entry before going to bed at night, or on the following day. Try not to wait longer than one day, however, as you might forget something important. Be totally honest in your diary; it is for your eyes alone. Even if what you find yourself writing down is disturbing, keep in mind that anything you can do to ease your headache problem is worthwhile.

After a few weeks, begin looking for patterns. You may not discover any, but it is more likely that you will. If these patterns involve problems with loved ones, try being more open and honest in your communication with them; you may want to consider going for counseling if necessary. If the patterns involve tension at work, this might be a signal to incorporate more relaxation exercises into your lifestyle and take stretching breaks, and to try to change your attitude on the job. On the other hand, the patterns you discover may involve physical habits, rather than emotions. For example, you might find you have headaches on the day when you spend more hours than usual at the computer terminal. This tells you to examine your posture, your lighting, and the setup of your chair and computer. The headache diary can be very effective in helping you identify those factors that are contributing to your headaches.

Chapter Three

Tension Headaches

"Remember those headbands that were popular in the seventies? When I have a headache it feels like I'm wearing one of those, only it's made of steel, and it keeps getting tighter and tighter," said James Q. Perhaps he chose this analogy because he is in the high-pressure fashion field. He spent most of his workdays hunched over his drawing table, working to meet his design deadlines. The emotional stress of his job, coupled with his strainful physical posture, conspired to make him a prime candidate for tension headaches.

Tension headaches, also known as muscle-contraction headaches, account for approximately 90 percent of the head pain people experience. These headaches may not be as debilitating or dramatic as other forms of headaches, but they can certainly make life miserable. Fortunately, tension headaches can usually be helped by holistic methods. Despite what you may have read or heard, there is no such thing as a classic tension headache "personality," unlike migraine "types." *Anyone* can get tension headaches; they seem to transcend all barriers.

In James's case, he needed chiropractic manipulation to adjust the restricted movement of his vertebral bones and deep muscle massage to release the chronic tension in his shoulders. Then he learned to take preventive measures. He moved his drawing table to a position that wouldn't cause him to hunch forward. During the day, he took breaks to massage his shoulders and neck and do gentle stretches.

"I thought job stress might be causing my headaches," said James, "but I wasn't about to give it up and go weave baskets in Woodstock or something. It was great to learn that I could relieve my stress and my headaches without sacrificing my work."

The Symptoms of Tension Headaches

Unlike migraines, tension headaches are not usually preceded by other symptoms. The pain may start first thing in the morning, or at any time during the day, although sleep is not usually interrupted. The headache may last only a few hours or as long as a few weeks; pain may be constant or ebb and flow.

The pain is usually dull and consistent, although in some cases it has a pounding, throbbing, or jabbing quality. In contrast to migraines, tension headaches are usually felt on both sides of the head, although they are occasionally one-sided. The pain is often felt as tight pressure around the head or neck. Frequently, the discomfort radiates down the neck from the head into the shoulders and upper back. These areas of the body often feel knotted, clenched, and uncomfortable.

Do You Have Tension Headaches?

The following quiz, like others in this book, has no right or wrong answers. It is designed to help increase your awareness and understanding of your headache problem so that you can pursue the best course of recovery.

- Do your neck, shoulders, or upper back often hurt when you have a headache?
- Do your neck, shoulders, or upper back feel stiff and tight when you have a headache?
- Are you often tense in your upper body?
- Do your headaches begin after spending a period of time in a position that strains or tightens your upper body?
- Does rubbing or massaging your head and/or upper body bring you any form of relief? Does relaxing help?
- Do you feel a viselike pressure around your forehead, scalp, back of head and/or neck when you have a headache?
- Does the pain start in the morning or during the day, rather than interrupting your sleep?
- Do your headaches often start after or during a period of great pressure?
- Do you feel that your life is highly stressful?
- Are you a perfectionist?
- Do you put great demands on yourself and/or people in your life?
- Do you take your job home with you, so to speak?
- Do you find it hard to relax?
- Do you often feel unhappy or emotionally distraught?
- Do you suffer from bouts of depression?
- Do you often try to hold your anxiety, anger, or frustration inside?

If you found yourself answering yes to any of the last nine questions, this is not a cause for shame or self-flagellation. It does not mean you are to blame for your headaches; nor does it mean they are "all in your head." Our world is extremely stressful, and it is hardly unusual to feel anxious, angry, frustrated, or depressed. You don't, however, have to be a helpless victim of these feelings and the headaches they can cause. You can learn ways to combat the physical effects of these emotions, to "de-stress" yourself.

If you are a classic tension headache type, try to keep in mind the axiom: "Health is wealth." What's the use of driving yourself hard to become successful if chronic headaches make it impossible to enjoy the fruits of your labor? Try to maintain a healthy balance between work and play in your life. Learn to let go of your job and truly relax during your leisure time. Remember that relaxation is replenishing and vital to your well-being.

If relationships are creating a great deal of tension in your life, take steps to make them more harmonious and fulfilling. It is beyond the scope of this book to discuss all the ways you can improve your relationships and your emotional life; however, there are many helpful volumes that deal with these matters. You might also consider professional counseling or joining a support group. It is not a sign of failure, weakness, or sickness to seek help; millions of healthy people find counseling a way to enrich their lives. Whatever method you choose, dealing with psychological issues may relieve some of your tension and the resultant headaches.

Perhaps, on the other hand, you are not particularly pressured, nervous, hard-driving, frustrated, worried, or depressed. This may well be. There are no hard and fast rules. People are individuals; each person has his or her own unique combinations of qualities and requirements. Even if you do not believe that you are the tension "type," however, you can most likely benefit from incorporating relaxation methods and other preventive measures into your lifestyle. Why? Because stress is an inevitable part of life and we are all prone to its physical effects.

What Constitutes Stress

Amanda G. was happier than she had ever been in her life. She was engaged to be married and was planning a big wedding. She and her fiancé were shopping for a house in the country. Recently, she had quit her full-time job in order to pursue a career as a free-lance writer. The assignments were coming in and the writing was going well. She couldn't understand why she was plagued with tension headaches during this wonderful period in her life.

When a friend suggested that the headaches might be stress-related, Amanda replied, "But I'm not tense, things are going great." Luckily, however, Amanda was open-minded enough to read some books on tension and stress reduction. She learned that stress comes in many forms and can be precipitated by happy events as well as unhappy ones. Willing to try almost anything to help her headaches, Amanda began practicing a simple form of meditation and also doing tension-relieving exercises. These practices enabled her to enjoy the exciting changes in her life without bothersome headaches.

You may think, "I'm not under stress, so I guess I don't get tension headaches." But this may be an erroneous assumption. Two researchers named Holmes and Rahl surveyed seven thousand people, charting their health in relation to important life events. From this research, they developed the following stress test, in which major life events are given a numerical value that represents the amount of stress they produce.

Check any events you have experienced within the last year and a half, then add up your scores. According to Holmes and Rahl, if you score over 300, you have an 80 percent probability of a change in your health. But even if you have a high score, that is no reason to think you are bound to become ill. A high score may be a helpful signal that you need to incorporate more relaxation into your life to counteract the effect of stressful events.

The Stress Test*

LIFE EVENT	VALUE	YOUR SCORE
Death of a spouse	*100*	
Divorce	*73*	
Marital separation	*65*	
Jail term	*63*	
Death of a close family member	*63*	
Personal injury or illness	*53*	
Marriage	*50*	
Fired at work	*47*	
Marital reconciliation	*45*	
Retirement	*45*	
Change in health of family member	*44*	
Pregnancy	*40*	
Sex difficulties	*39*	
Gaining new family member	*39*	
Business adjustment	*39*	

*Source: "The Social Readjustment Rating Scale" by T. Holmes and R. Rahl, *The Journal of Psychosomatic Research*, 11 (1967): 213–18.

LIFE EVENT	VALUE	YOUR SCORE
Change in financial state	*38*	
Death of a close friend	*37*	
Change to a different line of work	*36*	
Change in number of arguments with spouse	*35*	
Mortgage over one year's net salary	*31*	
Foreclosure of mortgage or loan	*30*	
Change in responsibilities at work	*29*	
Son or daughter leaving home	*29*	
Trouble with in-laws	*29*	
Outstanding personal achievement	*28*	
Spouse begins or stops work	*26*	
Begin or end school	*26*	
Change in living conditions	*25*	
Revision of personal habits	*24*	
Trouble with boss	*23*	
Change in work hours or conditions	*20*	
Change in residence	*20*	
Change in schools	*20*	
Change in recreation	*19*	
Change in church activities	*19*	

LIFE EVENT	VALUE	YOUR SCORE
Change in social activities	*18*	
Mortgage or loan less than one year's net salary	*17*	
Change in sleeping habits	*16*	
Change in number of family get-togethers	*15*	
Change in eating habits	*15*	
Vacation	*13*	
Christmas	*12*	
Minor violations of the law	*11*	

Many of these occurrences are unhappy events, which you would expect to cause stress. But some of the highly stressful situations may be a surprise because they are happy, positive events. What this test and the research behind it show is that "good" and "bad" events can be equally stressful and induce health problems.

Emotional stress results not only from negative events; it can also come from a positive change, such as an exciting new love affair, a promotion you've been looking forward to, an exotic trip, stepping up your social life, or participating in a new sport or hobby. Stress is an integral part of a stimulating, active lifestyle, and without it there would be stagnation and boredom. The holistic approach is not intended to eliminate stress from your life or curb the challenging activities you undertake. It is designed to help you get in touch with your body's response to stress and learn to restore a healthy equilibrium to your system before headaches develop.

In addition to the many varieties of emotional stress, other types of stress can affect your health. Physical stress can result from not getting enough sleep, performing hard physical labor, even overdoing sports or exercise. Physical stress can also result from injuries, structural imbalances, or any condition that prevents your body from functioning properly. Thermal stress can occur if you are subject to a sudden temperature change or a long period in an uncomfortable atmosphere. Chemical stress can occur if you eat food that you are allergic to, food containing chemical preservatives or too much sugar, from drinking, taking drugs, or smoking, and from exposure to pollutants and toxins in the atmosphere and water.

Whatever the causes of stress in your life, the end result can be a headache due to a complex series of physiological reactions.

The Fight-or-Flight Response

Tony S., an account executive in an advertising agency, is responsible for coordinating the work of the copywriters and artists, then presenting the advertising campaign to the client. Sometimes, a client responds negatively to a presentation that Tony has labored on for weeks; some of the clients are nearly impossible to please and make outrageous demands.

There are times when Tony has a tremendous urge to punch an unreasonable client. Of course, being a civilized man, he never does. In the past, he developed a tension headache instead. The difficult clients unwittingly activated Tony's fight-or-flight response.

Human beings, like other animals, have a natural,

built-in physical reaction to stress. Exposure to a threatening situation results in a series of physiological changes that prepares us to either flee or engage in combat. This response was vital for survival in primitive times, since it enabled a threatened person to run from a wild animal or swing a club at an unfriendly neighbor. Then, after the proper action was taken, the body could return to its normal state.

In modern times, however, the stressor (tension-provoking stimulus) can be something we have to face time and time again, such as a deadline at work or a traffic jam. Since we can't very well attack a demanding boss or run out of the car screaming, there is often no appropriate outlet for our physiological tension. Instead, the tension is held in the body and may result in problems such as headaches.

Unfortunately, the body cannot always distinguish between what is worth fighting for and what is not. Despite the innate wisdom of the autonomic and sympathetic nervous systems, they are unable to make value judgments when it comes to stress. They activate the fight-or-flight mechanism in situations when its response is not necessary for survival, and sometimes when we are not threatened at all.

LAS and GAS

Much of our understanding of the human body's reaction to stress comes from Dr. Hans Selye, a pioneer researcher and author. Before his work, many hypotheses had been made regarding the direct correlation between stress and physical malfunction, but Dr. Selye was one of the first to do definitive research on this topic.

Dr. Selye had a team of over one hundred researchers examine and test patients to determine what physiological changes took place within their bodies when they were under stressful situations. He discovered the important phenomenon that he termed the Local Adaptation Syndrome (LAS) and the General Adaptation Syndrome (GAS).

He learned that when we are under a certain type of stress—for example, emotional stress caused by arguing with a spouse—specific changes occur in our bodies, such as increased muscle tension and production of adrenaline. This is the local adaptation syndrome at work. If we are under thermal stress due to exposure to cold, LAS will speed up our metabolic rate to cause a rise in body temperature.

In contrast to the LAS, in which specific causes lead to specific changes, the GAS can be triggered by any type of stress and leads to a general adaptation response—physical changes throughout the body. While the LAS is often an appropriate response that protects us in some way, the GAS is often an inappropriate overresponse that can harm us.

The GAS is a three-stage reaction. The first stage, called the alarm reaction, is a mobilization of the body's defensive forces. During the second stage the body undergoes adaptations to the stressor. The third and final stage is exhaustion, during which the body mechanism handling the stressor breaks down. After this phase, the body may interpret preparation as being insufficient and muster all the forces once again, going back into the alarm reaction; this may perpetuate defensive measures that cause headaches.

The Physical Effects of Stress

Although the response to stress varies from one person to another, there is a typical series of reactions. Breathing becomes rapid and shallow, which increases anxiety and raises blood pressure. Heartbeat increases, pumping more blood to the brain. This leads to dilation (enlargement) of the blood vessels in the head, a condition that is present during migraines and sometimes in other headaches as well. Less blood is pumped to the extremities; hence the expression, "He's getting cold feet."

Blood flow is also shifted away from certain organs and glands, including the digestive tract, leading to the feeling of having "knots in the stomach." If this response continues, it can lead to food allergies and toxicity, which are frequently linked to headaches.

The hypothalamus, the "overseer" section of the brain, sends messages to the pituitary gland. The pituitary gland releases hormones that affect the endocrine system. The endocrine system governs the hormonal chemistry of the entire body. Think of the pituitary gland as a conductor and the endocrine system as an orchestra. If the conductor is off the beat, or if one of the instruments in the orchestra plays the wrong notes, the entire symphony is disrupted. It works the same way in your body. A disruption in any aspect of the endocrine system's functioning can have wide-ranging effects.

During the stress response, hormonal production is stepped up and altered, thereby upsetting the delicate balance of the endocrine system. Among other changes, the adrenal gland is stimulated, producing the "rush" of adrenaline that most of us have experienced. If the stress response continues over a long period of time,

The Endocrine (Hormone) System

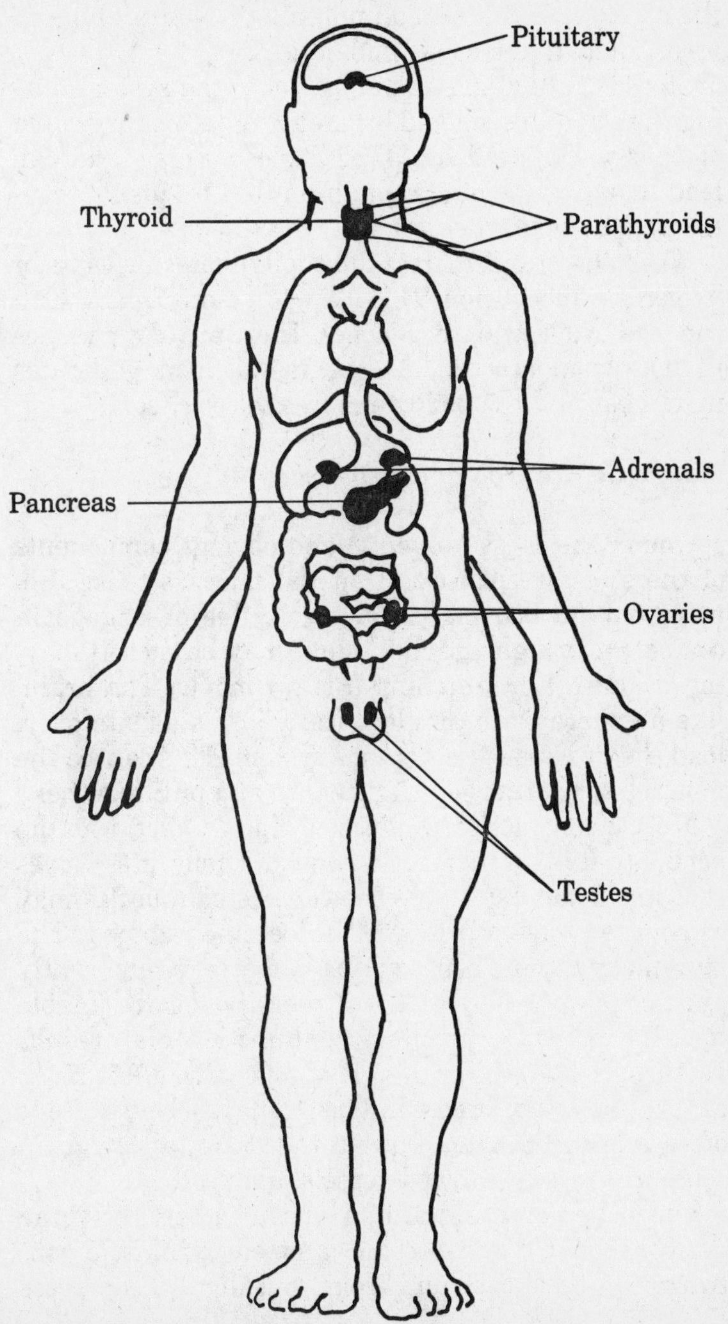

the result can be lowered immunity, low or high blood pressure, and hormonal imbalances.

Stored blood sugar is pumped into the system during the stress response. This creates a temporary spurt of energy, followed by lowered blood sugar, and can lead to hypoglycemia, a condition that frequently contributes to headaches.

When one is under stress the pupils dilate, allowing for longer distance vision. This allows in more light, which can lead to eyestrain headaches. There are also changes in body temperature, as the metabolism generates more heat and the body perspires to cool itself.

Muscle Contraction and Headaches

One of the most universal and obvious components of the stress response is that the muscles tense. Remember, the body is preparing to flee or engage in combat, although the individual may be merely having a quarrel or watching a scary movie. The brain, like a generator in an electrical plant, starts to overload the "wires"—the nervous system. This causes the muscles to contract—to tighten up and pull together.

Muscle contraction produces a ripple effect, like the pebble that is thrown into a pond and generates waves that reach the far shore. The contracted muscles may cause the bones of the skull to become jammed. The movement of these bones normally massages and gently pumps the pituitary gland; if these bones are unable to move properly, pituitary malfunction may result. Disturbances in the cranial bones can also affect blood circulation to the brain. In tension headaches, there is often a reduced blood flow to the brain, although in some instances the blood vessels dilate.

The bones of the cranium and also the vertebrae (the backbones) can become jammed by muscle contraction. The bones can become misaligned and press

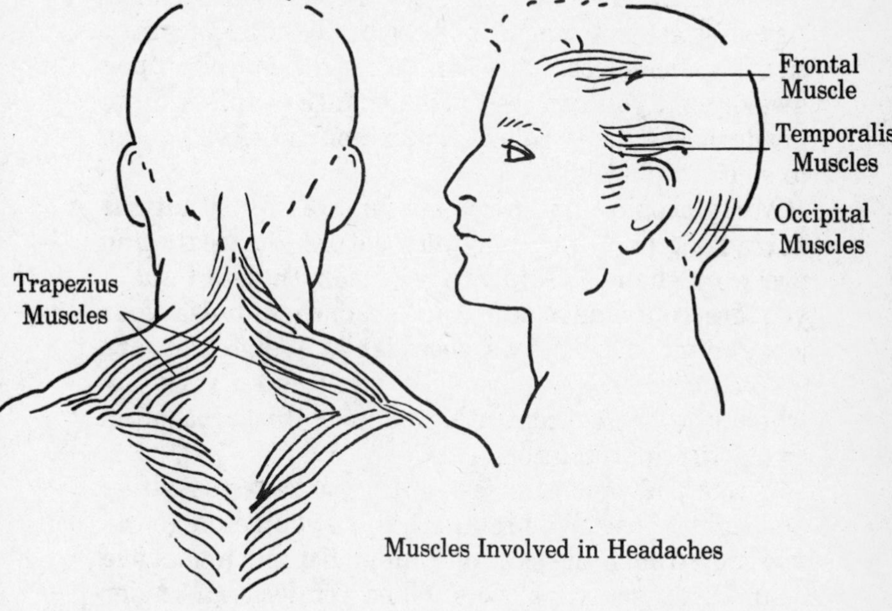

Muscles Involved in Headaches

on the nerves branching out between them. This upsets normal nerve functioning and often causes a pain signal to be sent to the brain and a headache to result.

/ The Temporalis Muscle /

The body is one integral unit, and any imbalance in it can lead to a headache. However, certain muscles are most frequently involved in headaches.

The temporalis muscle covers the side area of the head, extending from the temples down the front of the ear to the jaw. You can feel this muscle if you touch the area between your eyebrow and the top of your ear and clench your teeth. This is a spot where people often instinctively massage themselves when they have a headache, and with good reason. The temporalis attaches to the jaw and can tighten up when the jaw does. Many people grind their teeth and clench their jaws in their sleep, as a result of unrelieved stress and anger, or possibly because of nutritional deficiencies. This can cause a headache upon awakening; you can lessen the chance of this kind of headache by doing relaxation exercises before you go to sleep.

Many people tighten the jaw in stressful situations during the day; they may also eat too hurriedly and overwork their jaws during the meal. To determine if you are contributing to your headaches, tense your jaw and temporalis. Awareness is the first step toward correcting injurious habits. Do you tighten your jaw when you are concentrating? Touch this area often and notice its condition.

If you find that your jaw or temporalis is sensitive and tight, consciously relax and give yourself a gentle massage. Touch the skin in front of, behind, and above your ear for sensitive spots. When you locate a tender place, apply finger pressure to it for about ten seconds. Then release and find another spot that needs this treatment.

/ The Frontalis Muscle /

The frontalis muscle is in the region of the forehead and the front of the head. This muscle moves the eyebrows and the scalp. It is where people often place ice packs or rub themselves if they have a headache. It often tenses during periods of stress or deep concentration.

Once again, relaxation techniques help, and so does simple awareness. Try to become aware of the condition of this muscle throughout the day. Touch your forehead periodically to see if you are frowning or furrowing your brow. If you are, gently massage the frontalis, starting in the middle of the forehead and stroking outward toward the temples. Remember, you can think and work just as well with a smooth brow. You might prevent some wrinkles from developing, as well as a tension headache. The holistic approach often has unexpected side benefits.

Habitually squinting or frowning can cause the frontalis muscle to contract. Be sure you wear appropriate glasses or contact lenses and take care to have sufficient light and place your reading material close enough so you don't have to squint.

You might also try to release the neurovascular emotional points—two spots located at the top of your forehead, about three inches above your eyes. Close your eyes and apply a very light tugging pressure upward with your fingers to these spots. Hold them for about two minutes, then release. This technique is designed to relax your mind and body.

/ The Occipitalis Muscle /

The occipitalis muscle is located at the lower back of the head. Overcontraction of this muscle can lead to headaches. Other key muscles in this region link the skull to the neck and are involved in holding and moving the head. Contracted muscles in the neck area frequently contribute to tension headaches.

Chronic tension can develop in the neck muscles if you stand or sit with your head jutting forward, a very common mistake. Take a side view of yourself in the mirror to check your posture. There should be a slight forward curve at the top of your neck, but your head should not be thrust forward. If it is, try to lengthen the back of your neck and move your chin back. Lift the top of your head straight toward the ceiling. Don't do this to such an extreme that it feels tight or looks unnatural; a minor adjustment can make a great deal of difference.

Here is a little exercise to help you alleviate pressure on your neck muscles and develop a healthy posture: Imagine that a helium balloon, in your favorite color, is attached to the top of your head by a string. Visualize the balloon keeping your head floating effortlessly above your neck.

Many people develop tension headaches on the job, not only because of the psychological pressure, but also because of their physical working conditions. Take a few minutes to discover if your work habits may be exacerbating your headache problem.

Do you crane your head forward to type or work on a computer? Perhaps your work station needs to be rearranged so the tools are more accessible; maybe you need better light. Do you lean over your desk to read material? Position the reading material closer to you so you don't have to strain your neck. Do you hold the phone between your shoulder and your ear to free your hands? This very common mistake can lead to headaches by putting pressure on the muscles and nerves of your neck. Either hold the phone up to your ear, or, if you need to use both hands during calls, consider purchasing a set of lightweight headphones.

Many people hunch over to eat their meals. Try to bring the utensil up to your mouth instead of bending your head down toward the plate. Position your television set in a place where you won't be bending your head down to look at it. Some people get headaches when they play cards because they spend hours with their necks bent down toward their hands. Whatever you do, develop an awareness of your neck and try to keep it aloft. Mothers have the right idea when they tell their children to sit up straight!

When sitting up in bed, don't stuff pillows behind your head to prop it up. This may feel good temporarily, but it can cause neck constriction and headaches. Sleep on your side or back, never your stomach. Sleeping on your stomach forces your neck to be twisted in one direction for hours on end and can result in a headache upon awakening. Certainly you wouldn't want to spend three or four hours with your head turned all the way to one side when you're awake, so why do it when you're sleeping?

/ The Trapezius Muscles /

The large trapezius muscles begin at the base of the skull. They extend out over the shoulders in a triangular fashion, and down each side of the spine. Overcontraction of these muscles can affect the vertebrae, irritating the nerves and sending a pain message to the head.

Trapezius muscles can be chronically tense due to work conditions, living habits, bad posture, and stress. You can easily tell if your "traps" are tense by touching the tops of your shoulders. You can also check in the mirror. Do you wear your shoulders like earrings? Let them drop and relax. Do you carry a heavy shoulder bag? Try holding it in both arms in front of your body instead of burdening your trapezius muscles.

A certain amount of tension in the trapezius muscles is inevitable due to the demands of daily life. Stress certainly exacerbates this tension, however. Many people hold their anger or fear in their bodies. Whatever your situation, you can undoubtedly benefit from regularly doing exercises, self-massage, and relaxation procedures to relax this vital area.

In case all these different considerations sound overwhelming, remember that you don't have to take care of everything at once. Do what you can and make the changes you need to at your own pace. If you think it sounds like an awful lot of trouble, just consider what a hassle it is to have your activities disrupted by the pain. Isn't it worth it to make a few changes in your habits instead?

There are times, however, when correcting your habits and utilizing self-help methods is not enough. Professional help is often needed at the outset of a headache recovery program. Tension headaches can result from misalignments of the cranial bones and vertebrae, which require correction by chiropractic care. There also may be muscle tension that requires professional massage or physical therapy techniques.

Chapter Four

Migraines

Marisa M., a professional dancer, was fixing her makeup in a backstage mirror while she waited for her chance to audition for a nightclub revue. Suddenly, she couldn't see half her face: Her vision was obstructed by a series of dazzling, flashbulblike spots. She desperately wanted to stay and go through with the audition, but knew it was impossible.

Marisa stumbled outside and hailed a cab. Although her vision returned to normal during the ride, she knew the worst was yet to come. Soon after she was home, the migraine hit. It started as an aching throb on the left side of her face but soon enveloped her whole head. During the six-hour attack, she felt nauseous and achey, and had to run to the bathroom several times to vomit.

"I had migraines for six years, from the age of about eighteen. Sometimes a couple of times a month, sometimes a couple of times a week," said Marisa. "My social life was ruined because my dates couldn't understand why I would suddenly have to disappear into a dark room for hours. And my career—well, nobody wants to take a chance on a dancer who might be incapacitated in the middle of a performance. So I had to work two waitressing jobs just to pay the bills."

When the migraines first began, Marisa feared a

brain tumor and went to a doctor who did a series of tests to rule out that remote possibility. During the ensuing years, she had been given ergotamine compounds, which made her nauseous and also resulted in leg cramps. She was also given propranolol, a medication that caused her to gain weight and suffer from fatigue and gastrointestinal distress. "I tried a whole pharmacy of drugs," said Marisa, "but the side effects were horrendous. Also, it seems like they're always finding out that drugs that we thought were okay are really harmful, so I was really worried about taking them."

When Marisa went to a holistic doctor, he took a long look at her lifestyle. She didn't get enough sleep; she often stayed up all night worrying. She was judgmental and hard on herself; she never felt that she was good enough. Her diet was a shambles: She counted calories and practically starved herself to keep her weight down, yet indulged in candy bars and coffee.

Once Marisa learned precisely how her habits were contributing to her migraine problem, she was determined to change them. She cleaned up her diet, began practicing relaxation exercises that helped her sleep and also reduced her stress level, and started seeing a psychotherapist to deal with her emotional issues. These lifestyle changes diminished the frequency of her migraines, and, after about eight months, she ceased getting headaches altogether.

"Getting rid of my migraines was the motivating force that made me change to a healthier lifestyle, but now that I have, I feel better all over," said Marisa. "It's interesting . . . headache drugs had bad side effects on me, but the holistic approach has had only good side effects."

Do You Have Migraine Headaches?

Many people believe they are suffering from migraines when they are actually experiencing severe tension headaches. Yet migraines are distinctive for several reasons: They are vascular, involving fluctuations in the size of the blood vessels; and they usually involve symptoms in other parts of the body besides the head. The following quiz will help you determine if you suffer from migraines.

- Before a headache, do you experience visual disturbances, weakness, numbness, tingling, flushing, dizziness, swelling, nausea, diarrhea or an increased need to urinate, abdominal pain, and/or mental confusion?*
- Do you have a vague feeling of being unwell before a headache attack? Do you experience mood swings, food cravings, fatigue, or irritability prior to an attack?
- Do you have a history of migraines in your family?
- Do your headaches ever wake you from sleeping?
- Does the pain feel more intense on one side of your head than the other?
- Does the pain spread throughout the head, neck, and jaw? Do these regions feel sensitive to the touch?
- Is the pain deep and throbbing?
- Do you experience nausea, vomiting, diarrhea, or an increased need to urinate during a headache?

*These preheadache symptoms exist in only about 20 percent of migraine cases. The absence of these symptoms does not necessarily indicate that you do not have migraines.

- Do you feel abdominal pain or have a slight fever accompanying the headache?
- Do you feel chills, sore muscles, or achiness when you have a headache?
- Are you especially sensitive to light when you have a headache? Do you feel the urge to be in a dark, quiet room?
- Do you feel exhausted or have muscle aches for days following a headache attack?

As you can tell from this quiz, some of the chief distinctions that separate migraines from tension headaches are the symptoms that precede the attack and the disturbances in other parts of the body during it. There are no absolutes however, and some migraineurs (a French term for those who suffer from migraines) do not experience these symptoms. But if you *do* and if your headaches are debilitating and virtually incapacitating, most likely you suffer from one of the two types of migraine: classic or common.

Classic Migraines

The classic variety accounts for only about 20 percent of all migraines, but since they are so dramatic they receive a great deal of attention. What makes them so dramatic is the preheadache phase, which begins approximately ten to thirty minutes before the headache hits.

During the preheadache phase, a number of bizarre visual disturbances may occur. Migraineurs may see flashing spots, similar to those induced by flashbulbs, or zigzag patterns in neonlike colors. They may have a scotoma, an area of decreased or complete loss of vision, in one eye. Some people experience an episode of tunnel vision.

Premigraine disturbances of the senses are sometimes referred to as the "Alice in Wonderland Syndrome," due to the theory that some of Alice's adventures were inspired by author Lewis Carroll's symptoms. This syndrome includes distortions of the senses of vision, taste, and smell. The visual distortions sometimes resemble the effects of a fun-house mirror, but they are far from amusing.

Some classic migraineurs feel a mental confusion prior to an attack and may have trouble organizing their words or expressing themselves. Mood swings, exhaustion, mild fever, weakness, numbness, tingling, skin sensitivity, excessive sweating, abdominal pain, diarrhea, and the increased urge to urinate are some other precursors to classic migraines.

These symptoms usually fade within thirty minutes; then the head pain begins, often on one side of the head or around one eye. It then spreads as it gains in intensity. Moving the head often makes the pain worse, so victims may try to hold their heads still, with muscles taut. This can result in a muscle tension headache developing on top of the migraine.

In addition to the head pain, classic migraineurs often suffer from nausea, vomiting, abdominal pain, chills, and an overall feeling of pain and achiness in their bodies. The attacks can last anywhere from less than an hour to more than a day, and the victims may feel sore and tired for days afterward.

Common Migraines

This form of migraine accounts for about 80 percent of the cases. It does not have a distinctive preheadache phase, although some people may feel fatigue, lethargy, moodiness, irritability, or a drifting feeling of unease hours or even days before an attack.

The deep throbbing pain of a common migraine may shift in focus from one side of the head to the other, or may spread throughout the head and into the neck region. Victims are often hypersensitive to light, sound, and smells. As with classic migraines, vomiting, diarrhea and increased urination can accompany the head pain, and dehydration can result. Dizziness and mental disorientation are common. Cruelly, common migraine attacks can last as long as three to four days.

The Mechanism of Migraines

The exact causes and mechanisms of migraine headaches are not completely understood; however, researchers have found that the blood vessels of the head, face, and scalp play an integral role. During a migraine attack, the blood vessels initially narrow, or constrict. This reduces the blood flow to the brain and may be responsible for premigraine symptoms. After this constriction, some of the blood vessels widen, or dilate.

Many researchers believe that migraines arise from changes in the brain's chemistry that accompany the vascular fluctuations. Before a migraine begins, the level of serotonin in the body drops. Serotonin is a brain amine involved in regulating the size of blood vessels, sleep patterns, moods, and nerve-cell firing. Serotonin usually inhibits nerve impulses, so a reduced level may induce the brain to receive more pain signals. Neurokinin, a chemical irritant, is found to accumulate in the region of the blood vessels during a migraine attack. Prostaglandin levels in the bloodstream are believed to be a factor. Some migraine patients have also been found to have blood-platelet deficiencies.

Precisely what causes these vascular and biochemical changes is still open to debate in scientific circles. Researchers are now focusing on the role of the hypothalamus and brain function. Progress is being made, but we still lack a complete understanding of migraines.

You should not let this cause you to feel that migraines are an incomprehensible problem about which nothing can be done, however. A great deal is known about some of the causes of migraines and what can be done to prevent and treat them successfully. Let's take a look at some of these factors.

The Question of Heredity

Studies have indicated that between 70 and 90 percent of migraine patients had a parent, most often a mother, who also had migraines. Due to this high percentage, migraines are often characterized as an inherited disorder. Yet no one really knows whether inherited migraine tendencies are a result of genetic coding or learned behavior. In addition to genes, parents often pass on to their children patterns of dealing with emotions, relationships, and stress, all of which can have a major effect on headaches.

Although there is nothing you can do to change your genetic makeup, you are *not* doomed to endure migraines for decades if one of your parents did. You have the advantage of awareness and knowledge. You can take an honest look at your habits and emotional patterns to see if they are contributing to your problem. You can take advantage of healing methods that your parents may never have been exposed to. You can break the cycle of pain. But first you must decide that you deserve a pain-free life.

Sometimes people feel an unconscious guilt about accomplishing more than their parents, whether in the area of financial success, creative achievement, or personal happiness. They feel they should suffer as much as their parents did, that they don't deserve a better life. Take a deep look inside to see if this is one of your issues. If it is, you might consider undergoing some form of counseling to deal with it.

If, however, you can honestly say that you have no problem living a healthier, happier life than your parents, then you can let go of the fear that you will have endless migraines because they did. The holistic path offers you a wealth of resources to deal with your problem. Not only can you help yourself, but you may be able to help others. Perhaps you can pass on your knowledge and help your parents and children avoid suffering.

The Migraine Personality

Every day Abigail S. awoke at six A.M. so she would have a full hour and a half to groom herself before going to her job as an administrative assistant. She felt uncomfortable if her nails were chipped or her hair wasn't coiffed to her satisfaction. The other women in the air freight office didn't seem to care, but Abigail cared deeply about every detail.

This attention to detail made her a model employee. She was highly praised by her boss, and his approval was extremely important to her. She devoted herself to her work completely and kept the office meticulously organized, right down to the last paper clip. If there was still work to be done at five o'clock, she stayed until it was finished, often well into the evening. She simply could not bear it if all her tasks were not done to perfection. Abigail's apartment was as well ordered as her office: all the dishes washed as soon as they were used, every piece of clothing in its place in the closet. She liked feeling in control of her life.

Yet there was one aspect of her life that she couldn't control, and it caused her a great deal of anguish. About once a month, usually on Sundays, Abigail had a migraine attack. When a migraine struck, she would have to abandon whatever chores she had planned to tackle that day and spend it in bed. She hated the disruption of her plans almost as much as the pain. But she felt there was nothing she could do about it. She had been suffering from migraines since she was thirteen, and her mother had had them. Migraines seemed an inevitable part of Abigail's life, and she did nothing to seek relief.

Abigail's story provides a portrait of a classic "migraine personality": compulsively neat, organized, rigid, and perfectionistic. Migraine sufferers often lack self-esteem and so depend excessively on the approval of others. They are often workaholics and take on, with martyrlike resignation, more tasks than they can handle. Yet no matter how hard they try, they never feel good enough. They are usually afraid to express anger, fear, or frustration, and they keep their emotions bottled up inside.

There are no definitive statistics on how many migraineurs fit this personality profile. One Australian study showed that 25 percent of the migraine patients were obsessive perfectionists, but so were 25 percent of the general population. It may well be that migraineurs exhibit these traits to no greater extent than everyone else; it is impossible to say conclusively at the present time. Perhaps "migraine personality" is an unfair misnomer. If you *do* recognize some of the preceding characteristics in yourself, however, there is a chance that they are contributing to your migraine problem. Whether they are or not, you certainly owe it to yourself to seek help. These traits are usually rooted in childhood experiences, and you may need the expertise of a skilled counselor or psychotherapist to deal with them.

There are many types of therapy available, some of them short-term and goal directed. You might read a book on the different modalities to find out which one appeals to you, or contact your community mental health organization for suggestions. Your community organization may also be able to direct you to low-cost therapists if you are on a tight budget.

Try not to feel that it is shameful to seek help: Millions of Americans do it each year and benefit greatly. It is not a sign of being sick to go into therapy. Rather, it is a sign that you have enough healthy self-esteem to want to live a happier life and are willing to take action to achieve this goal.

Migraines and Women

Researchers estimate that between eight and twelve million Americans endure migraine headaches on a fairly regular basis. Although the ratio is nearly even in children who suffer migraines, adult female migraineurs outnumber adult males by a three-to-one ratio. A Danish study showed that approximately 20 percent of the women surveyed had at least one migraine attack by the time they were middle-aged. Other studies have concluded that 25 to 29 percent of women experience a migraine at some point in their lives.

And many of these women have migraine attacks daily or several times a week for years on end.

The attacks of over half of female migraine patients occur shortly before, during, or after menstruation, and approximately 14 percent have migraines while they are menstruating. Many women experience their initial attack around the time of menarche—the onset of menstruation in puberty. These patterns are probably due to the hormonal changes involved in menstruation.

The liver is involved with the breakdown of excess hormones during the menstrual cycle, and a toxic or sluggish liver can result in hormonal imbalances and headaches. A toxic colon can also cause liver malfunction. Embarking on a cleansing or detoxifying diet has helped many women overcome migraines as well as such cyclical ailments as premenstrual syndrome (PMS).

Most women who have previously suffered from migraines experience a worsened condition during their first trimester of pregnancy, but an improvement during the latter months. This improvement may be due to chemical changes, such as an increase in endorphin production. It has also been theorized that the mother's body may utilize the developing fetus's organs and glands to help her own body create positive chemical changes during pregnancy. Because of this phenomenon, some women state that they feel better than usual during their pregnancies, especially during the third trimester; however, their babies may be born with weaknesses and imbalances such as allergies, asthma, or blood-sugar-handling problems.

Menopause has a varied effect on the frequency of migraines. Some women have an increased number of episodes; in other cases the attacks diminish or cease altogether. This can sometimes be due to a weak liver that is unable to handle the changes in the body chemistry. The administration of estrogen either after menopause or after a hysterectomy can exacerbate preexisting tendencies toward migraines.

Birth control pills have been found to increase both the number of migraines and the intensity of the pain. Birth control pills frequently cause women who have never before had migraines to develop them and worsen the condition of those who had them before. The reasons include the estrogen influx and the vitamin deficiencies that the pills can cause. The pills can upset the body's delicate hormonal system, and an increased chance of migraines is only one of the possible risks involved in taking them. The convenience of birth control pills can be undermined by their possible side effects. Some migraine sufferers elect to switch to a form of birth control that does not interfere with the hormonal balances in the same way that birth control pills may.

Another thing women who suffer migraines can do is supplement their diet with multivitamins and additional vitamin B-6. Some clinicians have discovered that vitamin B-6 deficiencies can result from using birth control pills. A long-term deficiency of vitamin B-6 can interfere with proper functioning of the nervous system, possibly resulting in migraine headaches. However, toxicity may result from taking large doses of B-6 for a long period of time.

The Role of Diet

Joshua W., a middle-aged guidance counselor, had had frequent migraines since childhood. He took Elavil, an antidepressant, to cope with the depression that his migraines engendered. When he had an attack, he took a "headache cocktail," provided by a medical headache specialist. The potent combination of drugs would knock him out for four or five hours.

"It's part of my job as a guidance counselor to steer the kids away from drugs, and here I was taking them. I knew it was wrong," said Joshua. "So I was excited when I read that migraines can be caused by food allergies."

When Joshua went to a nutritionist, it was determined that he had hypersensitivities to eggs, milk, cheese, and wheat, all of which had been mainstays of his diet. When he eliminated these foodstuffs, and certain other foods known to be common headache triggers, he initially went through a withdrawal period, during which he had a terrible migraine. "I was just about ready to give up, but the nutritionist explained that I was undergoing withdrawal, just like someone would if they were withdrawing from drugs. She encouraged me to stay on the diet, and I'm glad I did." This withdrawal migraine attack was the last one Joshua ever endured.

A survey of three hundred leading headache experts found that most of them agree that dietary factors are involved in some cases of migraine, although they varied widely in their judgment of the percentage of cases affected by diet. Holistic practitioners feel that all headache sufferers should take their diets into consideration. By "diet" we mean everything that is consumed: all food, beverages, alcohol, recreational drugs, prescription medications, and over-the-counter remedies. Many medications can cause headaches; they should not be deemed harmless simply because they are prescribed by a physician.

While some foods are notorious headache triggers, individuals can also develop migraines because of allergies to substances that are safe for other people. Chapter Six includes a detailed list of trigger substances, as well as a method to determine hypersensitivities (allergies) you may have to certain foods.

Structural Problems

Migraines can result from many of the postural problems and work and personal habits that we discussed in the preceding chapter, "Tension Headaches." In case you skimmed that section because you are a migraine sufferer and thought it did not apply to you, we suggest that you go back and study it carefully. You need to be vigilant in your habits to ascertain that you are not allowing any structural problems to develop.

As we have emphasized, all parts of your health are interconnected and interdependent. Therefore, you must consider the functioning of every part of your body when dealing with your migraine problem. Migraines can stem from impingements of nerves, or misalignments or restricted movement of the spine or joints of the body. Imbalances in any area can have a ripple effect and alter the functioning of other parts of the body. A change in the fluid pressure within the skull, as well as altered blood flow to the brain, can be part of this ripple effect. Physically speaking, migraines are not necessarily "all in your head"; the underlying causes—as well as the effects—can, and often do, lie somewhere else in your body.

You can lessen the likelihood of structural problems contributing to your migraines by maintaining healthy posture and habits during all your activities, by doing gentle stretches, therapeutic movements, and relaxation exercises. By the time migraines develop, however, your structural problems may require professional attention. You may need to see a holistic practitioner to get your body back on the right track. Then you can keep yourself in shape with self-help methods.

Weather and Light

Some migraineurs find special significance in the expression "an ill wind." Changes in the weather seem to provoke their migraine attacks. These changes might be low-pressure fronts, increases in humidity, a drop in temperature, as well as the seasonal "ill winds" found in some regions.

No one completely understands the connection between headaches and weather, but many believe that it has to do with the physiological effect of ions in the air and also a change in the atmospheric pressure. Ions are subatomic particles that carry either negative or positive electrical charges; ion concentration may be partly responsible for the feeling of energy and well-being that being near water evokes. The ratio of negative to positive ions in the atmosphere changes as the weather does. If you feel certain that weather provokes your migraines, you might look into purchasing an ionizer unit for your home.

Migraine sufferers often become sensitive to light and seek out dark places during their attacks. In some cases, bright sunlight or flickering light seems to actually instigate the episodes. This can be due to weak adrenal glands, which cause the pupils to stay dilated too long, thereby letting in too much light. Weak adrenals can be caused by chronic stress or nutritional factors, so you may be able to strengthen them by performing relaxation exercises and by having a well-balanced diet with appropriate supplementation if necessary. As common sense would indicate, if you are light-sensitive consider wearing sunglasses and a wide-brimmed hat when exposed to bright light.

Weekend Migraines

Migraines often strike just when you are set to enjoy yourself, on a weekend or a holiday. This can be infuriating both to you and to your companions. But instead of complaining about the unfairness of life, let's look at what you can do to prevent this from occurring.

Do you drink a lot of coffee during the workweek and less on weekends? Coffee has an effect on the blood vessels; a sudden change in consumption can instigate a headache. But instead of dosing up on weekends as well as weekdays, we suggest that you kick the coffee habit altogether.

Your food or drink intake may also trigger weekend migraines. Do you eat more sugar, drink more alcohol or wine, or eat any unusual foods during your time off? The temporary pleasure of these indulgences is hardly worth the pain that may follow. Also beware of smoking or being in a smoke-filled room. You may be allergic to tobacco.

Altered sleeping patterns may also be a consideration. Sleep is a wonderful thing, but, like anything, too much of it can be detrimental. Oversleeping has been found to trigger migraines in some people. So if you are a weekend migraineur, try to stick with your normal sleeping pattern and wake up at approximately the same time you do during the week, unless you need to catch up on sleep.

You can experiment with these suggestions, see which ones apply to you and which ones help. Helping yourself beat migraines will probably mean making a few sacrifices, but nothing beats the pleasure of ridding yourself of headaches and enjoying a healthier life!

Chapter Five

Special Cases: Cluster, TMJ, Sinus, Eyestrain, and Environmental Headaches

HEADACHES COME IN MANY VARIETIES. IN THIS CHAPTER we will focus on types of headaches that are fairly widespread, although not nearly as common as migraines and tension headaches. It is important that those of you who do not suffer from "garden variety" headaches know as much as possible about your particular ailments so you can do as much as possible to alleviate them.

A Cluster Attack

After George J. finished work on the construction site, he headed, as usual, to his favorite local tavern. Sitting at the bar, he drank a couple of whiskies, smoked a few cigarettes, and joked with his buddies. George was a "man's man," down to earth, tough, decent. A tall, rugged fellow with blue eyes and thick blond hair, he was also popular with the ladies.

Through the haze of smoke and laughter, George became aware of an uncomfortable feeling of pressure in his left ear, similar to the feeling one experiences when an airplane descends. Then he felt a piercing pain around his left eye. The searing agony quickly spread, enveloping the left side of his forehead.

Soon George was overcome with excruciating pain. It felt as if the left side of his face was being stabbed over and over again with an icepick. His left eyelid drooped and his nose ran. George staggered out to his car, where he endured the rest of the attack, fighting a strong urge to drive his car into a brick wall and end his misery. Half an hour later, a time period that seemed like an eternity to George, the stabbing sensations began to lessen in frequency and finally subsided altogether. But the relief was only partial, since George knew that he would probably have another attack that night, or the next day. He went back into the bar to drown his sorrows.

Do You Have Cluster Headaches?

Although less than one percent of the population is estimated to have had at least one cluster episode, 85 percent of this group are men. Ninety-four percent of them have been found to be heavy cigarette smokers and 91 percent are moderate to heavy drinkers.

Even if you don't fit this profile, however, you may have cluster headaches. The following quiz will help you determine if you do:

- Do your headaches usually occur during a one- to three-month period, followed by a period of remission?*
- During your "bad" periods, do you usually have at least one and up to six attacks per day?
- Is the pain concentrated on one side of your face?
- Do you have sinus congestion or a runny nose on one side during an attack?

*Some people endure chronic cluster headaches with no remission period, but these cases are rare.

- Does your eyelid droop and your eye tear on the painful side?
- Is the pain intensely piercing, burning, or throbbing?
- Do you feel the urge to strike out, bang your head, pace wildly, or shout out during an attack?
- Do the episodes last about fifteen minutes to one hour?

As you might gather from this quiz, attacks usually occur during a one- to three-month period; hence the name "cluster." This headache period is followed by a period of remission, which can last anywhere from a few months to many years. There are variances to this pattern, however, and some cluster headache victims endure attacks all during the year or at random intervals. People usually experience the first attack during their twenties or thirties, but again, this varies.

The most outstanding characteristic of cluster headaches is the excruciating pain, which has been described as being one of the worst agonies imaginable. The attacks usually begin rather suddenly, build in intensity to a high level, then taper off or stop completely after fifteen minutes to two hours. The pain is usually located on one side of the head, in the area of the eye, temple, and forehead. It is so intense that its victims are sometimes driven to striking out violently, banging their heads, or even thinking of suicide.

There are usually secondary symptoms on the affected side during an attack. The nostril often runs or becomes congested. The eyelid sometimes droops, and the eye tears. The skin may become flushed and sweaty. Yet these symptoms are nothing compared to the searing pain.

Causes of Cluster Headaches

During a cluster headache attack, the blood vessels widen, which is why clusters are grouped with migraines under the label "vascular headaches." In fact, cluster headaches are referred to by several other names, including "episodic migrainous neuralgia," "Harris's neuralgia," and "Horton's headaches."

Since vasodilation occurs during cluster attacks, it is thought that certain ingested substances that cause blood vessels to dilate might be triggers. Food allergies are probably a factor, since histamine, a body chemical that is released when the skin or membranes are exposed to an allergen, is found in the tissues during an attack.

Drinking alcohol can precipitate an attack, as can eating foods to which you are allergic or that affect the blood sugar level, such as sweets, tea, coffee, soda. Simply not eating frequently enough or not eating sufficient quantities of food can instigate an attack. Foods that contain nitrates, such as hot dogs and other packaged red meats, are to be avoided. Nitrate is also found in dynamite and can cause headaches in workers who are exposed to it.

Treating Cluster Headaches

The intense level of pain makes cluster sufferers especially desperate to alleviate their misery. They often turn to prescription drugs for relief. The frequency of the attacks induces some patients to overmedicate themselves. Adverse side effects are more likely to occur because of the amount of drugs taken.

Recently some medical doctors have started prescribing lithium for their cluster patients. This potent drug, which is often given to manic-depressives, can create toxic conditions in the kidneys and affect thyroid functioning. It can be especially hazardous to cluster victims who, due to the extent of their suffering, take more than the recommended dosage.

A safer treatment is the inhalation of pure oxygen from an oxygen mask, which has been found to help some people during the course of an attack. A preventive measure is to keep your diet free of nitrates and to try to determine if you have any food allergies. It is best to avoid cigarette smoking and smoke-filled rooms. Sleeping regular hours and avoiding napping may help.

Above all, it is imperative to avoid drinking *any* alcohol during the cluster period, and to cut down on alcoholic intake all year round. This may sound like a tall order, one that is difficult to fill, but the hellish pain of a cluster attack should provide motivation.

As with all forms of headaches, those who suffer from cluster headaches should be examined to determine if there are underlying causes, such as structural imbalances or chemical or emotional problems.

TMJ Syndrome Headaches

The temporomandibular joint (TMJ) is formed by the mandible (jawbone) attaching into a groove in the temporal bones (the right and left bones of the skull). If you place your fingers in front of your ear while moving your mouth, you can feel the TMJ. Muscles attached to the mandible enable us to chew and speak.

Malfunction of the temporomandibular joint is referred to as TMJ syndrome. Symptoms of this syndrome can be an inability to open the mouth widely or discomfort upon doing so, clicking and popping noises when the mouth opens and closes, pain radiating from the jaw, neck pain, and headaches. Keep in mind, however, that many people with TMJ syndrome do *not* experience pain in the jaw. Some people have major malfunction of the TMJ without accompanying discomfort, while others endure chronic pain.

The pain caused by TMJ syndrome is usually felt on one side of the head, although some people feel it on both sides. It is concentrated in the areas in front of the ear, cheek, and temples, although the neck and shoulder muscles may also be affected. The pain can range from a dull ache to stabbing spasms. It is sadly ironic that it can be aggravated by activities that are normally healthy and enjoyable: eating, talking, laughing. Stress and tension can also be aggravating factors. Some people clench and grind their teeth while sleeping as a result of stress. Many people endure chronic symptoms on a daily basis for many years, without realizing that the TMJ is causing these problems.

When there is an imbalance or restriction in the TMJ, it can cause a chain reaction. If the temporal bones in the skull do not have a full and balanced range of motion, the other bones of the skull may not move properly. The membranes attached to the inside of the skull can become twisted. The blood supply and fluid balance in the skull can be affected and chemical changes can occur in the brain and nervous system. Headaches may be one of the end results.

Do You Have TMJ Syndrome?

Although it is often overlooked, TMJ syndrome is actually quite common. Since there are conflicting definitions and diagnoses of this problem, exact figures are hard to come by, but the American Dental Association estimates that sixty million Americans may have TMJ symptoms. The majority of the victims are women in their twenties, thirties, and forties.

The following quiz may help you discover if your headaches are related to TMJ syndrome:

- Do you experience pain in the areas around your ears, the side of your face, and your temples?*
- Is there an aching sensation in your jaw, especially after eating or talking?*
- Is the area around your TMJ tender to the touch?
- Is it difficult for you to open your mouth wide without feelings of discomfort or limitation?
- Do you usually hear loud cracking, clicking, or popping noises when you open your mouth or chew?
- Do you grind your teeth at night?
- Do you tend to tighten or clench your jaw when you are under stress?

What Causes TMJ Syndrome?

The precise causes of TMJ syndrome are the subject of great dispute among health professionals and researchers. Many dentists believe that TMJ syndrome is due to malocclusion (misalignment of the teeth and jaw), which causes the jaw muscles to overcompensate and become tense and tired. They may treat the syndrome with splints and bite plates to correct the bite. While this works for some patients, this approach fails for many others because it often ignores the underlying structural imbalances that may be contributing to the problem.

There are theories that TMJ syndrome results from an inherent weakness in the jaw region. The preponderance of women who suffer from this problem has led to speculation about hormonal imbalances being a

*Although pain in these areas is a sign of TMJ syndrome, this problem can exist even if no pain is present.

factor. Traumatic injuries to the jaw region are another possible cause.

Stress and tension tend to exacerbate the pain involved in TMJ syndrome. Grinding the teeth during sleep or clenching the jaw during the day can be manifestations of anxiety, unresolved anger, and fear.

The Holistic Approach to TMJ Syndrome

While holistic practitioners often take all the aforementioned elements into account when treating TMJ syndrome, they are also aware that all parts of the body are interconnected and dependent upon each other. A problem in the TMJ can result from a pinched nerve in the neck or from imbalances in the pelvis and/or other areas of the body. Therefore, it is necessary to work to balance the entire body in addition to the TMJ itself. Sometimes it is helpful for a team of holistic professionals to work together.

Vivien W. developed TMJ syndrome when she was in law school. It started with feelings of tightness in her jaw and pain in her neck. "I guess I should have done something to nip it in the bud, but I felt I was too busy to bother," she said. After a few months, she started to feel muscle spasms and pain around her ear, along with frequent headaches.

When Vivien couldn't ignore the pain any longer, she went to see her doctor. He diagnosed her as having TMJ syndrome and sent her to a dentist. The dentist did extensive work to correct her bite and gave her a splint to wear. Still, the pain and headaches persisted.

"My husband told me I would sometimes grind my teeth during the night, and I knew I was tense during the day, what with law school and all. I felt it was my fault that I had this TMJ problem, that it was because

I was too uptight. This made me mad at myself, and of course that only made everything worse," said Vivien.

After six months of finding little relief from the dental work, Vivien tried the holistic approach. Since tooth-grinding can be due to a calcium and magnesium deficiency, she was placed on a program of vitamin and mineral supplementation. She learned about the importance of getting enough rest and eating a healthy diet so she could cope with the demands of her lifestyle. She explored relaxation methods to help relieve her anxiety.

"I wanted an instant miracle cure, and at first it was hard for me to accept that making these long-range changes would really help. But after a year of TMJ pain, I was about ready to try anything," said Vivien.

Work was done to release the restrictions in Vivien's cranial muscles, balance her cranial bones, and realign her cervical spine. She continued to see the dentist, who made adjustments to her splint as her TMJ began to realign. After about five months, her structural problems were corrected and her TMJ began to function properly. The TMJ pain and headaches began to subside. "I still get a twinge now and then, but now I know what to do about them and I don't feel so helpless," said Vivien.

TMJ syndrome is a multifaceted problem, and no practitioner can guarantee success. If you suffer from TMJ pain and related headaches, however, trying the holistic approach is likely to help you.

Self-Help for TMJ Syndrome

If you have TMJ syndrome, you should be especially careful to treat yourself well. Get enough rest. Eat a well-balanced diet of natural foods and chew your food thoroughly. A vitamin and mineral supplementation program that includes calcium and magnesium can be helpful. Avoid putting physical pressure on your jaw and neck. Exercise regularly, but try not to tighten your jaw or neck during your workout. Many people with TMJ syndrome find swimming a highly therapeutic form of exercise. Include gentle, careful stretching in your fitness regimen, paying particular attention to your neck and shoulder muscles. When you are in a stressful situation, touch your jaw to see if you are tensing it. If you are, try to relax. Remember, it's safe to let go. It's very helpful to use relaxation methods regularly to reduce tension and the stress it places on your TMJ.

Massage can sometimes help reduce TMJ pain and headaches. You can massage yourself, but it is also a pleasant luxury to have someone do it for you. Apply finger pressure for about ten seconds to each tender spot around your ear. Take hold of your ears and gently pull them out and down (away from your head). Rub behind and in front of your ear, then up to your temples.

Using massage oil, stroke downward on your neck. Massage only the sides and the back, never the front of your neck. Massage along the sides of your neck vertebrae and up to the skull. Press on the sensitive points where your neck vertebrae meet the skull. Also massage the muscles on both sides of your mandible (jawbone). Use thumb pressure to find tender spots in these areas, then press on them for ten seconds. You can also place your hands on both sides of your mandible and gently pull it down. Hold for twenty seconds, then release.

Sinus Headaches

A sinus headache involves a feeling of pressure and throbbing pain around the eyes, forehead, temples, and cheekbones. This is usually accompanied by a runny or congested nose and teary eyes. Since similar symptoms can result from a migraine or tension headache, sinus headaches can be difficult to self-diagnose.

Although we all have sinuses, few people know exactly what they are or what they do. The sinuses are air pockets within the layers of bone on both sides of the nose and forehead. The mucous membranes, which line the sinuses, secrete mucus. The mucus is meant to flow through the small spaces in the sinuses, down into the nose. If these spaces are blocked, the fluid builds up, creating a feeling of pressure and pain. The blood vessels in the mucous membranes dilate as the membranes become inflamed.

Relieving Sinus Headaches

There are cases when sinus problems are due to calcification of the tissues or a deviated septum, making surgery necessary, but these instances are unusual. Sometimes pinched nerves or other structural problems can lead to sinus blockage. Most commonly, the blockage is caused either by an infection or an allergic reaction.

Whenever Teresa L. had a headache, her nose felt stuffed and her eyes were runny. Since her symptoms seemed to match those of the actors on the television commercials, she swallowed the sinus headache remedies they were selling. These medications usually made her feel better, partly because of the aspirin they contained and partly due to the placebo effect. She was unaware that both the aspirin and the caffeine in these medications were contributing to her frequent stomachaches.

Teresa went to see a nutritionist not because of her headaches, but because of her abdominal pains. The nutritionist recommended that Teresa stop eating all dairy products. When she did this, not only did her stomach feel better, but her headaches ceased. Her sinus problems and the resulting head pain were due to allergies to dairy products.

An allergic reaction to dairy products is a very common cause of sinus problems. Dairy products often produce increased amounts of phlegm and mucus, creating blockage in the sinuses. Whether you have sinus headaches or not, you are probably better off without dairy products, since they are one of the most common allergens. You can get the calcium you need from green leafy vegetables, nuts, grains, and supplements, instead of from dairy foods.

Sinus problems can also result from allergies to wheat, corn, peanuts, tomatoes, apples, or oranges. If you suffer from sinus headaches—or any type of headache—we recommend that you try to determine if you have any allergies by using the techniques described in the next chapter (see pp. 81–99).

If you have a sinus headache, treat yourself to some self-massage therapy. Begin by rubbing in the grooves on both sides of your nose in a circular motion for thirty seconds. With your thumbs, steadily press in the hollows where the top of your nose meets your browbone for about ten seconds. For the next thirty seconds, massage above the center of your eyebrows in a circular motion.

Locate two spots called the lymphatic reflexes in the hollow just below the collarbone, where it meets the breastbone. These spots may be sensitive and tingly when you rub them. Using three fingers of your right hand, massage your left lympathic reflex for about thirty seconds in a circular pattern. Using your left hand, do the same for your right side. These reflexes, when stimulated, often cause the sinuses to drain. Try to do this entire sequence about six times a day when your sinus headache is in its acute stage. However, be mindful that prolonged or recurrent sinus inflammations or infections require professional evaluation.

Eyestrain Headaches

It seems glaringly obvious that eyestrain can cause headaches, but sometimes the last thing we think of is the simplest. Eyestrain headaches are usually caused by contraction of the muscles around the eye. The symptoms are similar to those of tension headaches.

When is the last time you had your eyes examined? Eyes are constantly changing, and even people who have good vision may need correction as they get older. And if you wear glasses or contact lenses, it's a good idea to see a professional regularly to make sure your prescription is right.

An ophthalmologist specializes in eye diseases and can determine if your headaches are due to glaucoma or another serious malady. An optometrist primarily prescribes lenses, but can also uncover the existence of certain diseases. An optician supplies the lenses and frames. It's worthwhile to make regular visits to skilled, caring practitioners. When it comes to your health, it doesn't pay to look for bargains.

If you wear contact lenses, make sure you clean them carefully and use the enzymatic protein remover once a week, and that you have the lenses replaced periodically. Eyestrain can occur if you are allergic to any of the chemicals in the lens-care solutions you use. Many people are allergic to the preservatives which are found in some solutions; manufacturers now offer thimerosal-free solutions "for sensitive eyes."

Eyestrain headaches can also result from poor lighting. If the lighting flickers or is too weak or too bright, eyestrain can develop. By providing a light that more closely imitates nature's, full-spectrum lighting can alleviate eyestrain and also the "seasonal depression" that some people experience. Sunglasses with polarized lenses and wide-brimmed hats can reduce the possible eyestrain that can result from bright sunlight.

If you work for long hours on a computer, looking at the screen might cause eyestrain headaches—as well as tense muscles from poor posture. You might alleviate both problems by taking breaks and by purchasing a screen that reduces glare.

Give your eyes the rest they need. If you get headaches from too much reading, try to pace yourself accordingly. Take periodic breaks to close your eyes and relax them. Try a very restful technique called "palming." First, remove any corrective lenses you may wear and turn down the lights. Place your hands over your eyes so your palms block out all light. Then look into the blackness for about thirty seconds. Close your eyes and lower your hands, then open your eyes slowly after a few seconds.

For some temporary eyestrain headache relief, you can do a little self-massage. Never rub directly on your eyes. Instead, press up on the eyebrow ridge with your thumbs, moving from the top of your nose to the outside of your eyebrows. Stroke in gentle circles around your eyes. Massaging your forehead and temples can also help.

Headaches During Sex

Some people suffer tremendous pain at their moments of peak pleasure. This is called benign orgasmic cephalalgia, meaning a severe headache at or near the time of orgasm. This happens most often to individuals who have a history of migraine headaches. The attacks strike suddenly and last anywhere from minutes to hours. Although usually harmless, as the name suggests, benign orgasmic cephalalgia can signal a serious illness. Therefore, we recommend that anyone experiencing "orgasm headaches" go to a health professional for a complete examination.

Headaches during sexual activity may also stem from muscle contraction due to unusual strain being placed on the neck and shoulders.

If you have sex-related headaches, it is important to consider the possible psychological ramifications. Are you relaxed or tense with your sex partner? Do you harbor guilt feelings about sex? Guilt can make you feel that you deserve to be punished, that you deserve pain. Are you unconsciously looking for an excuse to avoid sex? Headaches can be a way to avoid many activities, including sex. We are not implying that all sex-related headaches are due to unresolved issues regarding sexuality, but it is necessary to consider all the possibilities.

Environmental Headaches

Getting headaches at work may indicate not only job tension but also an unhealthy environment. Many large office buildings do not have a free flow of fresh air. The chemicals and pollutants in the building can be sealed in, thereby becoming more likely to cause headaches. Some of the possible dangers are: asbestos or formaldehyde used in construction or insulation; toxins in the heating or air-conditioning systems; ozone emitted from copying machines; secondary cigarette smoke; chemical cleaners; and pesticides.

There are no easy answers to the problem of a "sick building." You can improve the environment somewhat by installing electronic air cleaners, however. If the building allows it, simply opening the windows to provide fresh air circulation might help. You can enlist your coworkers to lobby the management to make whatever changes are necessary to clean up your office environment.

Your home should also be well ventilated. Too much heat, especially when cheap heating fuels are used, can create a headachy, fatigued feeling. Opening the windows every so often can solve this problem, as can making sure that your air conditioners or fans are clean and not spreading allergens around your home.

If you or someone you live with smokes, you might get an air filter machine to clean the air. Some people who live in highly polluted areas find these air-cleaning machines useful regardless of whether or not there is a smoker in the home.

Toxic chemicals, such as asbestos and formaldehyde, are often used in home construction and insulation. Chemicals in cosmetics, cleaning agents, paints, or linoleums can be headache triggers. Aluminum cookwares and plastic dishwares or utensils can cause allergic responses, including headaches. Overexposure to lead, carbon monoxide, and benzene also can cause headaches.

There are no simple solutions to the problem of environmental headaches, because it may be impossible for you to avoid some of the culprits. What you *can* do is try to limit your exposure to toxic chemicals as much as possible. Study your surroundings to see if there are any health hazards and, if necessary, take steps to create a healthier environment. You might help your colleagues and family as well as yourself.

CHAPTER SIX

The Role of Nutrition

ARE ANY OF THE SUBSTANCES YOU CONSUME CONTRIBUTING to your headache problem? It is highly likely that the answer to this question is yes. Hypersensitivity to specific foods and liquids contributes to an enormous number of headaches. There is some controversy over the exact percentage of headaches caused by diet; however, from a holistic point of view, careful and healthy eating is a prerequisite for well-being.

The Digestive System and Toxicity

In order to understand how ingested substances can trigger headaches, let's take a look at how the digestive system functions.

When you take a bite of food, digestive enzymes in your saliva begin to break down starches. The food travels down a long tube, called the esophagus, which goes from the mouth into the stomach. In the stomach, digestive chemicals are produced to break down the food further. From the stomach, food passes to the small intestine, where additional chemical changes occur and food particles are broken down into smaller units (carbohydrates, fats, proteins, vitamins, miner-

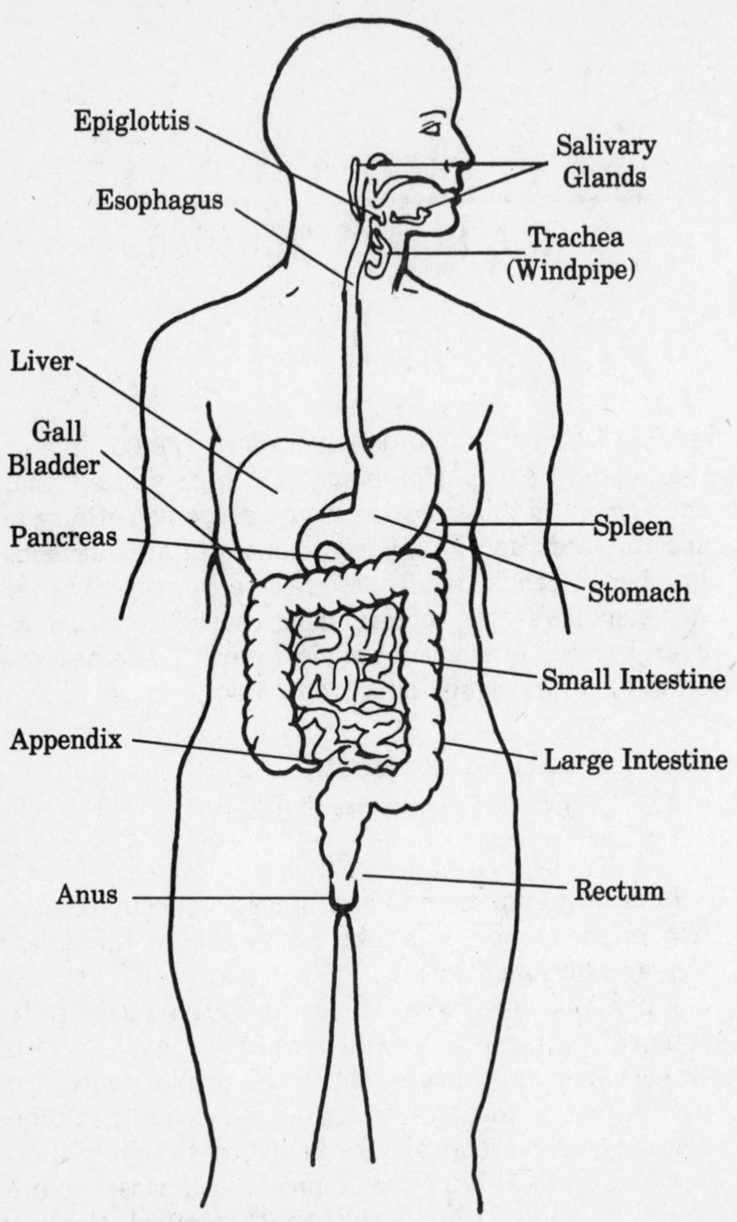

The Digestive System

als, waste, etc.). The particles that can be utilized by the body are transported through the walls of the small intestine into the bloodstream. The bloodstream carries these substances to different parts of the body, where they are used as fuel for proper functioning and material for repairing weakened areas.

The substances that the body cannot use are meant to pass from the small intestine into the large intestine and be eliminated from the body by way of a bowel movement. However, if unhealthy substances are ingested, or nutritional deficiencies exist, or if there is malfunctioning of the digestive system, problems can occur.

The waste material can build up in the large intestine and begin to putrefy. The large intestine can become a virtual toxic dump of poisonous material. Some of this material can be reabsorbed into the bloodstream, causing the blood to become toxic. When the liver tries to clean the blood, the liver can become toxic. This, in turn, can lead to endocrine (hormonal) imbalances and blood sugar problems, potentially causing symptoms such as headaches.

Some of the substances that can cause toxicity are:

- Medications
- Recreational drugs (marijuana, cocaine, etc.)
- Alcohol (including wine and beer)
- Cigarettes, pipe tobacco, cigars
- Pesticides sprayed on fruits and vegetables
- Rancid oil in snack foods
- Hormones injected into cattle and poultry
- Food that has been improperly refrigerated or stored and is partially spoiled

The first step toward detoxification is to eliminate toxic substances from your life. If this seems overwhelming, try to give up one category each week.

Remember that there are always choices. You can replace toxic substances with healthy ones. Here are some of the alternatives:

- Utilize natural healing methods instead of medication whenever possible; check with your doctor first.
- Practice relaxation exercises instead of drinking or taking drugs.
- Substitute fresh fruit juice, seltzer, or spring water for soda or cocktails.
- Enjoy an array of herbal drinks instead of caffeinated beverages.
- Buy organically grown fruits and vegetables or grow your own, if possible.
- Purchase a health food cookbook so you can learn to prepare convenient fresh dishes instead of relying on frozen or packaged goods.
- Munch on nuts, seeds, or hot-air-popped popcorn instead of packaged snacks.
- Eat soyburgers instead of hamburgers or hot dogs.

Candida Albicans

Jill M. was always exhausted and drowsy at work. She also had irritable bowel syndrome—stomach pains, constipation, and diarrhea. But her worst problem was migraine headaches. "I could struggle through my day with the other things, but when a migraine hit, I had to give up. And they hit every few weeks."

Jill's ailments were caused by food allergies. The food allergies were a result of an overgrowth of candida albicans in her system. Candida albicans is a yeast fungus that is always present in the body, with its level usually kept in check by helpful bacteria. When people take antibiotics or other drugs, this "good" bacteria is destroyed along with the "bad" bacteria responsible for the illness. This can allow the candida albicans to grow unchecked. Sweets, alcohol, wheat, and foods containing yeast can also make candida albicans flourish.

Jill went on a diet that eliminated all products containing sugar, dairy, yeast, wheat, and fermentation. She avoided high-sugar fruits, and vegetables in the nightshade family (tomatoes, eggplants, bell peppers, and potatoes). "It sounds like a tough diet, but I'd been so miserable for so long, I was determined," said Jill. She ate primarily fresh poultry and fish, rice, millet, oats, and a variety of fresh vegetables. Supplements of vitamins, minerals, hydrochloric acid, acidophilus, and antifungal nutrients were also part of her recovery program.

"After a couple of weeks my stomach began to calm down, I had more energy, and the migraines hit less often. After about four months, the migraines stopped completely. And I even lost this extra ten pounds I'd been carrying around for ages. So I look better as well as feel better," said Jill.

Candida albicans has now begun to be recognized as a widespread health problem. It is often an underlying reason for food allergies, which often cause headaches. A qualified nutritionist or holistic doctor can determine if you have candida, and help restore your system to a balanced state.

Food Allergies

Food allergies occur when your body is unable to break down a food or drink properly. A series of unhealthy chemical and functional responses follow and can cause a host of complaints, including headaches.

Any food or drink containing a substance to which you are allergic can trigger an adverse reaction. The following substances have been found to be common allergens:

- Caffeinated drinks (coffee, tea, colas)
- Alcohol
- Drugs
- Tobacco
- Chocolate
- Sugar
- Dairy products (including eggs)
- Food preservatives, additives, and colorings
- Citrus fruits
- Barley
- Wheat
- Rye
- Corn
- Peanuts
- Onions
- Nightshade vegetables (tomatoes, potatoes, peppers, eggplants)
- Shellfish

You will notice that some foods on this list are normally considered healthy. Each person has a unique internal environment, and food allergies are highly individual. Just as different cars need different types of fuels, so do human beings. What is perfectly safe for your friend may cause you to have a headache. Some detective work is necessary to discover your particular food allergies.

The Food Elimination Program

The food elimination program is a way for you to learn which foods cause allergic reactions for you. It requires a good deal of willpower, but getting rid of headaches should provide adequate motivation.

It has been suggested that for the first five days of an elimination program, you eat *only* combinations of the following:

- Brown rice
- Millet
- Rice cakes
- Fresh fish (not shellfish)
- Turkey
- Tofu
- Beans
- Lettuce
- Spring water

After five days, you may begin to introduce foods back into your system one at a time. Eat a food for one day, then stop and see how you feel for the next two days. Use a notebook to keep track of which food you have added and your reactions. If you feel okay and don't experience any headaches, you can keep this food in your diet. Then experiment by adding another food.

Here's an example of how this program works: For five days you eat only the foods listed. On the sixth day, you add whole wheat bread to your diet. On the seventh and eighth days, you don't eat bread, but you feel fine, so you know that you can continue to eat whole wheat bread. On the ninth day, you drink milk. You get a headache the following day. This means it is likely that milk is a food you should avoid.

Sample Food Diary

DAY	*FOOD ADDED*	*REACTION*
1	Apples	none
4	Tomatoes	none
7	Swiss Cheese	headache later that night
10	Corn on the Cob	none
13	Whole Wheat Bread	headache next day
16	Milk	headache next day
19	Chicken	none

Conclusions: Likely allergies to cheese, milk, and other dairy products, and products containing wheat

It's best to use your common sense and not reintroduce substances that are basically unhealthy, such as chocolate and tobacco. If you find that you seem to be allergic to something that is normally safe, such as wheat or corn, you can retest this food. It may be a coincidence that your symptoms appeared, so retesting the food about a week later might give you a clearer picture. Even though you test positive to a certain food, it is recommended that you retest the substance approximately every three months. It has been found that when some people get healthier and their bodies are functioning better, they no longer react to food to which they were once allergic.

Finding Professional Help

If the food elimination program seems too daunting, there are alternatives. You can keep a journal of what you consume and when you have headaches and look for patterns. Or you can visit a health professional, such as a holistic doctor or nutritionist, to help you pinpoint your particular food allergies and also determine if you have problems with candida albicans or hypoglycemia. A health professional can design a diet and a vitamin/mineral supplementation program that is customized for your specific needs. It can be much easier to overcome your digestive disorders with this type of guidance than if you do it all on your own.

At this time, there is no formal license examination or required schooling for nutritionists. There are, however, many educational programs and seminars that train individuals in nutritional counseling. Be certain to check out a practitioner's educational background before you submit to his care. Seek recommendations from other patients and from other health professionals. A referral from a holistic medical doctor or chiropractor can help ensure that the nutritionist you see is qualified and skilled.

Migraine Triggers

Migraine sufferers should be particularly careful to avoid substances containing high levels of certain amines, which can cause vascular and chemical changes that trigger an attack.

These substances include:

- Cheeses
- Alcohol (particularly beer and red wine)
- Foods containing yeast
- Pork, game, and organ meats; smoked, aged, and packaged meats
- Chocolate
- Citrus fruits, figs
- Cream, sour cream, yogurt
- Pods of lima and navy beans and peas

- Vinegar
- Herring, caviar, smoked fish
- Pickled and fermented foods
- Flavor enhancers, particularly MSG

Ultimately, it is up to *you* what substances you do or do not consume. We're not presenting this information to take away your freedom to eat what you wish, but to enable you to make educated and informed choices. Keep in mind that even if you eliminate toxic substances, migraine triggers, and allergens, there is still a wide world of food for you to savor.

Basics of Healthy Eating

A lifelong program of healthy eating and drinking will make you less susceptible to most health problems, including headaches. Basic guidelines are that about 15 percent of your food intake should come from fish, poultry, dairy, and eggs (unless you are a vegetarian or have food allergies); 30 percent from fruits and vegetables; and the balance from grains, seeds, nuts, and beans. Try to avoid red meat, as cattle are often fed an excess of hormones and antibiotics to help them grow.

It's not just what you eat, but when, that matters. Odd as it may seem, it's healthiest to eat your biggest meals early in the day. Start with a large breakfast, have a medium-sized lunch, then a light dinner. Nibble on two or three snacks of vegetables, fruits, or nuts during the day. Just as water can clean the outside of your body, it can also clean the inside. Try to drink at least eight glasses of spring water a day. Seltzer, flavored with a little fruit juice if you wish, is a good alternative to soda.

Try to avoid canned and processed foods that contain chemical additives that can trigger headaches. Enjoy the fresh flavor of raw, unprocessed, uncooked, "live" foods: vegetables, fruits, nuts, and seeds. Eating live foods will help you feel more alive! When you wish to cook vegetables, steam or pressure-cook them for only a few minutes so they retain their nutrients.

Red meat contains chemicals that can trigger migraines, so introduce yourself to some healthier protein alternatives: raw nuts, beans, and tofu. Fish is an excellent protein source, although canned fish and shellfish may contain high levels of toxins from pollution. If you're in the mood for meat, try to buy organic or range-fed poultry instead of the ordinary variety, which often has additives and hormones.

Carbohydrates can be quite healthful, except those containing white flour, a headache trigger in some individuals. Brown rice, barley, buckwheat, bulgur, millet, quinoa, and whole grain cereals, pastas, and whole wheat bread are smart choices.

Manufacturers are now required to list ingredients. This makes it easier to maintain a healthy diet. Before you buy a packaged food, study the label for such ingredients as sugar, salt, preservatives, and flavor enhancers like MSG. These artificial flavor enhancers can easily be replaced by using fresh herbs. Skillfully used, herbs can create many delightful tastes.

Salad bars are proliferating around the country and can be very convenient for busy working people. Before you dip in, check with the management to make sure they don't spray preservatives on the salad bar. Then choose the fresh offerings instead of the canned goods.

You can still maintain your nutritional integrity when you dine out. Most high-quality Chinese restaurants will refrain from using MSG if you request them to. Order dishes that are described as steamed, poached, baked, or fresh. Bring along an herbal tea bag so you can forgo the coffee, and try to resist the sugary desserts. Use mealtimes as a chance to relax. And *bon appetit*!

If you would like to learn more about good nutrition and healthy eating, there are many excellent books to guide you. We have listed some of them in the "Suggested Further Reading."

Vitamins and Minerals

It's best to get as many vitamins and minerals as possible through a balanced, natural diet. Few people's diets consistently provide them with a full range of essential nutrients, however. This is true, in part, because modern agricultural, shipping, storage, and cooking methods can rob food of vitamins and minerals. Toxins such as recreational drugs, medications, alcohol, and preservatives can also interfere with the body's ability to absorb food nutrients. Therefore, it's a good idea to take supplements to avoid possible deficiencies.

Most inexpensive supplements are made from synthetic materials, so it's better to spend a little extra and purchase products made from natural food sources. Megadoses can be helpful for certain health problems, but should only be taken under the supervision of a professional. If you are taking them on your own, choose low-dosage, sustained-time-release supplements to avoid overloading your system.

A good basic regimen is as follows:

- A multivitamin/mineral after breakfast
- B-complex, vitamin C, vitamin E, and a chelated multimineral after dinner

Birth control pills deplete B-6, so an extra fifty milligrams with your multivitamin is advisable if you're on the pill. B-6 can also help relieve premenstrual syndrome and related headaches. Inositol and choline are two other B-vitamins that are especially helpful for headache sufferers. Pantothenic acid, another member of the B-family, can relieve stress. Tryptophan is an amino acid that has natural tranquilizing effects. Soy-based protein tablets can help offset a protein deficiency. Acidophilus and fiber are helpful to regulate the digestive system. Many nutritionists suggest that their patients supplement their diets with betaine hydrochloric acid and pancreatic enzymes to help with conditions such as candida and food allergies.

Herbal Medicine and Homeopathy

Herbs were the original medicines, and their recorded use stems back to ancient Egypt. Throughout the ages, herbal medicine was used extensively by Far Eastern, Middle Eastern, and North and South American Indian practitioners, as well as Western folk healers. The "back to nature" movement of the 1960s and 1970s revived interest in herbal medicine in the United States.

For relieving headaches, herbalists recommend teas and capsules with a slew of different ingredients. Many books on herbal medicine describe these remedies, which can afford pain relief in some cases. However, herbal medication can have one of the same drawbacks that popping artificial painkillers does: It deals with symptoms, not causes. You may feel some temporary pain relief, but since the underlying causes have not been corrected, your headaches are likely to recur. For this reason, we believe that herbal medicine should be incorporated into a holistic treatment program under the guidance of a professional, rather than be used as a temporary panacea.

Homeopathy was developed in the 1800s by Samuel Hahnemann, a German physician. It is based on the principle that "like cures like": a substance that produces a symptom when taken in a large dose by a healthy person can cure that symptom when taken in a diluted form by an unhealthy person. This is similar to the concept behind vaccinations.

Homeopathic medicines may be helpful for some illnesses. Some homeopathic remedies contain herbs that can induce toxic reactions or temporarily exacerbate symptoms, however, so we advise against self-administration. It is better to deal with the causations of your headaches than to stifle the pain with medicines, even natural ones.

Hangover Headaches

A night on the town can mean an aching head the next morning. One of the reasons for the ubiquitous hangover headache is that drinking alcohol depletes vitamins and minerals and causes dehydration. A preventive measure is to drink several glasses of water and take a multivitamin before going to sleep.

In the morning, drink several more glasses of water and some fruit juice and have a nutritious breakfast. If you have the luxury of time to sleep off the hangover, a relaxation technique might help you fall back asleep.

The Ice Cream Headache

After tasting a delicious ice cream cone, you may experience a flash of pain in your throat, followed by a headache. The so-called ice cream headache can actually occur when any ice-cold substance is ingested: The sudden chilling of the mouth sends a pain message through the nerves. This can usually be avoided if you eat cold substances slowly and carefully. Be aware, however, that ice cream can lead to headaches for another reason: hypoglycemia.

Hypoglycemia

When Barbara A. woke up at three A.M., her throbbing headache and nervous thoughts kept her from falling back asleep for hours. She awoke the next morning with a headache, dreading the day ahead. After gulping some aspirin along with her morning cup of coffee, she went to her job as a legal secretary.

Tired and unable to cope, she felt a wave of anxiety when her boss handed her a routine contract to type. At lunchtime, she had a bagel and a cola, then coffee and ice cream for dessert. When her boss pointed out a few errors in the contract she had typed, she felt like crying. Soon her head began to throb.

When Barbara went to see a holistic doctor, it was determined that she had hypoglycemia—low blood sugar. This common and often undiagnosed condition can cause emotional responses such as nervousness, mental confusion, poor memory and concentration, fits of anger, irritation, and depression. Other symptoms include interrupted sleeping patterns, fatigue, craving for sugar and/or caffeine, a rapid pulse, and muscle pains. Among the most prevalent and recurring symptoms are headaches.

The body has a vast network of blood vessels that transport blood, oxygen, nutrients, and glucose (blood sugar) throughout the body. Foods are broken down during the digestive process and converted into pure glucose. Glucose is the fuel that allows many parts of the body, including the brain, to function. The level of glucose in the bloodstream is carefully monitored by the pituitary, thyroid, and adrenal glands, the pancreas, and the liver. They work to maintain the appropriate glucose level in the blood at all times. For instance, during exercise, the organs and glands raise the amount of glucose in the blood to ensure that the muscles are properly fueled and don't become fatigued.

Eating foods containing sugar or consuming toxic substances such as alcohol, tobacco, caffeine, marijuana, or cocaine causes a rise in the glucose level in the blood. The brain then signals the pancreas to produce insulin. The insulin helps the glucose cross the blood vessel walls into the tissues of the body. This leads to a temporary "rush," or feeling of energy. However, if you continue to take in those substances, the pancreas becomes oversensitized and produces too much insulin. Too much glucose crosses from the blood vessel walls into the tissues, and the blood glucose (sugar level) drops.

When the glucose level in the blood drops, an alarm goes off in the body, since the brain will die if it doesn't get enough glucose to its cells. A complex chain of events occurs, causing the glucose level to shoot up. This roller coaster effect puts an enormous strain on the body and can even lead to diabetes (high blood sugar).

Help for Hypoglycemics—and Everyone Else, Too

Like so many other causes of head pain, hypoglycemia can be controlled by following the basic rules of good nutrition. It's of primary importance to significantly reduce the intake of foods containing sugar. Remember that there is sugar in cereals, white bread, condiments, sweetened fruit, juices, and sodas, as well as in the more notorious cookies, candies, cakes, ice cream, and chocolate.

Here are some tips for beating the sugar habit:

- Don't keep any sweets in your home. If you have to run out and buy something sweet, you may think twice before eating it. Don't use the rationalization that the sweets are for the other family members; everyone is better off without them.
- Eat a small portion of fresh fruit, nuts, seeds, or raw vegetables when you have a sugar craving.
- Keep a sugar diary. When you long for something sweet, write down what you are doing and how you are feeling at that moment. This may tell you something about the psychological dynamics behind your craving.
- Try a brief exercise or self-massage break when you start thinking about eating a sugary snack.
- Artificial sweeteners can increase your longing for the real thing. They can also have harmful side effects, so try to avoid them.
- Carry your own nourishing snacks when you are traveling in order to avoid vending machine sweets.
- Keep some nutritious treats in your desk at work so you can indulge yourself without eating sugar.

Let's see how Barbara, whom we mentioned earlier, fared under this system. At first Barbara thought it would be very hard to give up sugar, but it soon became easier when she began to cultivate awareness about what she was eating and its effect on her body. When she started to think carefully about her choices, she began to make the right ones. She learned to satisfy her sweet tooth with fresh fruit.

The most difficult step for Barbara in her recovery program was to give up coffee. Caffeine has an addictive quality, and when people give it up they often experience a low-grade headache that can last a day or more. Barbara was going to take some aspirin when this occurred, until she was informed that many painkillers actually contain caffeine. Instead, she used relaxation techniques to help her through the withdrawal period. After she was freed from her addiction, she no longer needed coffee as a stimulant. She felt more energetic and alert, as well as less nervous, all day long.

Many people experience nervousness, irritability, muscle twitching, rapid heartbeat, gastrointestinal problems, hemorrhoids, and toxicity, as well as headaches, from caffeine consumption. Caffeine is found in many soft drinks, painkillers, and diet aids as well as coffee, tea, and chocolate.

There are many healthy alternatives to caffeinated beverages. Coffee substitutes are available in health food stores; they are made from such ingredients as bran, wheat, barley, and molasses. There are a myriad of herbal teas that provide variety and good taste without caffeine. Flavored seltzers or pure fruit juices are a refreshing replacement for soda. Try to avoid "decaffeinated" beverages, which are often processed with harsh chemicals that linger.

If you really need a lift, ginseng can provide both mental and physical stimulation. It can also help you assimilate vitamins and minerals, instead of robbing your body of them as stimulants do. Ginseng is available in capsule form, liquid concentrate, as a tea, or in root form. The root form was used by Cherokee Indian medicine men in their ancient healing rituals to treat headache sufferers.

Barbara also began to increase her intake of protein, a good idea if you suspect hypoglycemia. She started to eat six small meals a day instead of three large ones, in order to keep her blood sugar level balanced. Supplements of the mineral chromium, also known as the glucose tolerance factor, helped stabilize her blood sugar level.

When Barbara changed her dietary habits, she experienced an enormous change in her life. She slept soundly and could cope with stress on the job more easily. No longer jittery and easily upset, she performed better at work and enjoyed it more. Her manner became more pleasant and calm, which created new and better relationships with people. And headaches no longer plagued her days and nights.

Hypoglycemics often find it difficult to tolerate even small amounts of alcohol, tobacco, marijuana, cocaine, and other drugs. Avoiding hypoglycemic headaches is only one of many important reasons to give up these substances. Many books and treatment programs offer help in kicking these habits. Don't be afraid to seek help—you have nothing to lose but destructive addictions.

It's easier to give up a negative habit if you replace it with a positive one. When you feel the need for a cigarette during work, get up and stretch instead, or give yourself a little neck massage, or drink a glass of water or juice. Instead of going for a drink to relax after work, exercise or meditate to unwind. Meditation and breathing exercises also provide a feeling of euphoria and well-being. Be imaginative and discover the many ways you can indulge yourself and feel wonderful without harming your body.

Chapter Seven

Mind Over Headache

YOU MAY HAVE NOTICED A RECURRENT THEME IN THE holistic approach: the importance of relaxation. Relaxation is the antidote to stress. Relaxation techniques help you get in touch with your body and increase your control over your physiological functions. Although these techniques will not alleviate all the tension in your life, they can substantially reduce the physical effects of stress. They can help reduce the frequency and intensity not only of tension headaches, but also of migraines and most other types.

There has been a recent escalation in research on how mind techniques can combat illness. In 1980, Robert Adler coined a name for this growing field of study: psychoneuroimmunology, or PNI. PNI researchers have found that relaxation techniques, combined with creative imagery, affect brain wave patterns, blood pressure, respiration, gastrointestinal function, hormonal and neurotransmitter levels, the nervous system, and the immune system. Patients suffering from a host of ailments, from cancer to insomnia to back pain to headaches, have been helped by mind techniques. Studies have shown that relaxation and imagery can reduce chronic pain as well as strengthen the immune system, which helps defend the body against disease. By using relaxation techniques, you can improve your immunity and overall health as well as help your headaches.

The Relaxation Response

When we use the term "relaxation," we are not alluding to such pleasant activities as watching television, sharing a meal with a friend, or sitting in the sun, therapeutic though they may be. Rather, relaxation refers to techniques and practices that invoke a series of specific physiological changes called the relaxation response.

The term "relaxation response" was coined by Dr. Herbert Benson, a prominent Harvard cardiologist, researcher, and author. The relaxation response counteracts the stress response. During the relaxation response, the activity of the sympathetic nervous system slows down. There is a reduction in the level of catecholamines, neurotransmitters that are connected to the stress response. The number of breaths per minutes decreases, the heart rate slows, and the blood pressure level drops. Yet there is increased blood flow to the brain, which can help prevent headaches.

During the relaxation response, brain waves become less random and more synchronized. More alpha brain waves are produced, creating a feeling of calm. Muscle tension decreases, and the body goes into a self-healing state. Since the brain controls the proper functioning of the body, evoking the relaxation response can have tremendously positive effects on both the mind and body.

Unfortunately, the relaxation response does not happen automatically, as the stress response does. According to Dr. Benson, in order to enjoy the benefits of the relaxation response you must put yourself into a different state of consciousness. You will learn that this is not as far out or as difficult as it may sound. There are simple ways to alter your consciousness so that your mind and body enter a state of deep relaxation.

We will teach you a variety of the relaxation techniques so that you can try whichever ones appeal to you. Remember, anything new takes some getting used to, so it may take you a few attempts to experience the full benefits of these techniques. Once you do, you can decide which work best for you and incorporate them into your lifestyle. Most likely, in addition to helping your headache problem, they will also enhance your outlook on life.

Deep Breathing

Deep breathing is one of the most basic relaxation techniques. Breath is life, and the quality of our breath alters the quality of our lives. How we breathe has an enormous effect on our mental and physical well-being.

Recognition of the importance of breath is far from new. Devotees of yoga have practiced deep breathing for many centuries. And most people have been advised to "Take a deep breath" before attempting a difficult task. Still, many of us have forgotten how to breathe properly. Since breathing is an automatic function, we tend to take it for granted.

Did you ever notice the way a baby or a person in a deep state of sleep breathes? The abdomen gently rises and falls. This is because they are breathing into their diaphragms and not merely into their chests. The air is drawn into the diaphragm area, then the rib cage and lungs, and finally the chest. We were all born to be diaphragmic breathers, but many of us get into the habit of breathing shallowly, only into the chest. Breathing into the diaphragm allows for more efficient inhalation of oxygen and exhalation of carbon dioxide.

Another principle of deep breathing is to breathe through your nose, rather than through your mouth. Have you ever heard the admonition, "The nose is for breathing, the mouth is for eating?" There is a scientific basis for this saying. The nose is marvelously constructed for breathing. It contains little hairs, called cilia, which serve as air purifiers, sweeping out debris in the air as you inhale. Since the mouth contains no such safeguards, more impurities and pollutants are inhaled if you breathe through it.

Don't try to sniff the air in with your nostrils when you inhale. Let the impulse come from deeper inside. It may take you a while to get this, but you will recognize that you are doing it correctly because it will feel deep and comfortable. Many people exhale by blowing the air out of their mouths, but again, it is better to let the part of your body that is built for breathing do the work. Of course, there may be times when your nose is congested and it is difficult or impossible to breathe through it, but under normal circumstances, breathing through your nose should become a habit.

You can practice deep breathing for relaxation purposes by lying down with a small pillow under your head, lying flat on your back, or sitting in a comfortable, upright position. Loosen your clothing and take off your belt so your body feels unrestricted. Close your eyes and your mouth. Remember, all deep breathing is done through the nose.

Always begin by exhaling completely. Inhale deep into your diaphragm. Think of your abdomen as a balloon that you're trying to fill up with air. To check that you're breathing into your diaphragm, place your hands on your abdomen. You should feel it rise up as your diaphragm expands. Continue to inhale, filling up your rib cage, your lungs, and finally your chest. Hold the breath in for a few seconds, then exhale, also through your nose, as slowly as you can. Exhale completely and feel your stomach contract as you do so. Repeat the complete breath at least ten times.

As the deep breathing becomes more comfortable, start counting the duration of your breaths to yourself. Counting has two benefits: It encourages you to inhale and exhale longer, and it helps clear your mind of other thoughts. When distracting thoughts pop into your mind during deep breathing, try to let them go without giving them much attention, and return your focus to your breath and counting.

Inhale for eight counts, hold for four, then exhale for eight. You may find it difficult to exhale for this long. If so, temporarily shorten the duration of the breath holding. Try to control your exhalation so you don't let the breath out in one big huff. When you are comfortable with the 8:4:8 ratio, you can change the pattern. Inhale for eight counts, hold for four, exhale for twelve. Another variation is to inhale for twelve counts, hold for six, then exhale for twelve. Make the breaths as long as possible without any strain.

Deep breathing is very calming, but it is also energizing, since it bathes the cells with fresh oxygen. It is possible to get up from a five-minute deep breathing session feeling as refreshed as if you had an hour-long nap. Obviously, this is a highly convenient relaxation technique, since you can breathe anywhere, anytime.

When you are feeling stressed out at work, a few minutes spent on deep breathing might prevent a tension headache from developing. If necessary, you can keep your eyes open; no one will know that your mind is on your breath and not your work. If you are angry at your spouse, a deep breathing session can alleviate the tension. When you feel confused or overwhelmed, whether for personal or professional reasons, deep breathing can help clear your thoughts. Even when you are in the throes of a headache, deep breathing can make it easier to cope.

Alternate Nostril Breathing

Another breathing method that can help headache sufferers is alternate nostril breathing, a yoga technique. Actually, breathing is usually dominated by one nostril or the other. For a period of one to over three hours, we breathe mainly through one nostril, then switch over to the other side. This pattern may reflect which side of the brain is most active. It may affect the functioning of our circulatory and nervous systems. Definitive research remains to be done in this fascinating field; however, it has been demonstrated that alternate nostril breathing has a calming effect and helps some people reduce the pain and frequency of headaches.

To practice alternate nostril breathing, sit up straight and comfortably. Close your eyes and focus on your breath. Rest your left hand in your lap and use your right thumb to cover your right nostril. Inhale slowly through your left nostril, for a count of eight. Then uncover your right nostril and use your right pinkie finger to block your left nostril. Exhale slowly for a count of eight through your right nostril. With the left side still covered, inhale slowly for a count of eight through your right nostril. Then switch fingers, blocking off the right nostril, and exhale for a count of eight through your left nostril. Do this cycle at least six times.

This may sound complicated, but it's not. Just remember to switch nostrils on the exhalation and to exhale for at least as long as you inhale. As you become more advanced, your exhalation can be longer than your inhalation. You will probably find that on some days it is very difficult to breathe through one nostril or the other, while on other days it is relatively effortless. If you enjoy this exercise and find it beneficial, you can do it for up to ten minutes a day.

Autogenic Training

Around the turn of the century, Oskar Vogt, a physiologist specializing in the study of the brain, found that some patients reduce their tension, fatigue, and headaches by inducing a state of self-hypnosis. In the 1930s, psychiatrist Johannes Schultz noticed that when his patients were under hypnosis they experienced a pleasurable feeling of warmth and heaviness. The warmth was a result of blood vessel dilation. The heaviness was due to muscle relaxation. These discoveries prompted Schultz to develop the relaxation method known as autogenic training. Autogenic training is a way to learn to gain control over your physiological functions, as well as to relax.

When you first begin autogenic training, it is easiest to do so lying down. Later, when you are more experienced, you can do it sitting up, which makes it a "portable" method like deep breathing. Choose a dimly lit but well-ventilated room, where you will not be disturbed by a telephone or by other people. Loosen your clothing and take off any jewelry or glasses you might have on. Lie on a mat, carpet, or blankets on the floor, or on the bed if you have a very firm mattress. Place a small pillow under your head, or lie flat. Your legs should be slightly apart. You can place a small pillow under your knees if it will make you more comfortable. Your arms should be relaxed, down at your sides but not touching your body. Make sure your weight is evenly distributed. Your position should be as relaxed and limp as possible.

Close your eyes and take a few deep breaths. You are going to concentrate on making the following suggestions to yourself.

/ Autogenic Suggestions: /

1. My right arm feels heavy and warm.
2. My left arm feels heavy and warm.
3. My right leg feels heavy and warm.
4. My left leg feels heavy and warm.
5. My abdomen feels relaxed and warm.
6. My chest feels relaxed and warm.
7. My heartbeat is steady and calm.
8. My breathing is deep and relaxed.
9. My back feels heavy and warm.
10. My shoulders feel heavy and warm.
11. My neck feels heavy and *cool.*
12. My head feels heavy and *cool.*

Take a few more moments to let yourself float on a feeling of well-being. Then say to yourself, "I feel completely relaxed and refreshed." Slowly open your eyes and stretch your arms and legs. Arise slowly and try to spend the next few minutes in a low-key and pleasant manner.

Before you try this technique, try to memorize the suggestions. Say each phrase silently to yourself two times. Pause as long as it takes to feel the suggested sensation in between phrases.

When you first start your autogenic training, it may be difficult for you to experience the suggested feelings and sensations. Don't become frustrated or get angry with yourself if this happens. There is no such thing as winning or losing, or being right or wrong when it comes to relaxation. Give the technique a chance if you think you can benefit from it;

try it every day for a week or two. Most likely it will become second nature. If you keep trying and still can't invoke the autogenic suggestions, then perhaps another relaxation technique would suit you better.

Progressive Relaxation

In 1929, Dr. Edmund Jacobsen first described his success in treating tension headaches by using a technique he called progressive relaxation. Progressive relaxation is now one of the most widely used stress-reduction techniques. It is a way to perceive fully the difference between tension and relaxation in your body. This method helps you become aware of when and where there is tension in your body, so you can relax before a headache sets in. This exercise is preventive, not curative. It should be done when you are feeling normal, rather than when you have a headache.

Begin by lying down comfortably in a quiet, dimly lit room. Remove any restrictive clothing, and close your eyes. Follow this sequence of exercises:

1. Inhale and hold your breath; clench your right fist and stiffen your right arm while you lift it. As you exhale, drop your arm and hand and let them completely relax. Repeat on the left side.
2. Inhale and hold your breath; point your right toe and tighten your right leg while you lift it. As you exhale, let your leg flop down and relax. Let it be soft and heavy. Repeat on left side.
3. Inhale and, while holding your breath, tighten your abdominal muscles. Exhale and let your abdomen relax.
4. Inhale and hold your breath; tense your shoulders and upper back, lifting them off the floor. Exhale and drop your shoulders and upper back, allowing them to feel very open and relaxed.

5. Inhale and lift your head off the floor about five inches. Exhale and let your neck completely relax. The neck is especially important for headache sufferers to relax, so give this one some extra time. Let your head sink into the floor, let your neck feel very long and relaxed.
6. Inhale and, holding your breath, pucker and tighten up your face. Exhale and let your face open up and relax.
7. Repeat to yourself: "My entire body is relaxed. I am filled with a sense of calm and well-being." You may want to rub your hands over any part of your body that still feels a remnant of tension. When you feel ready, get up slowly.

Try to bring the awareness created by this exercise into your daily life. Stay in touch with the state of your body. When you feel a particular area getting tense, try to relax it. This can help prevent chronic muscle tension and the headaches that may result from it.

Overall Body Relaxation

The following relaxation exercise is an excellent way to alleviate tension in your body and relax your mind at the same time. This exercise can be done any time you have ten minutes to lie down. It is safe to do even when you are in the throes of a headache. Many people enjoy doing it directly after they get home from work in order to dispel the tensions of the day quickly.

Read the instructions through several times until you have them memorized and then say them to yourself, or make your own relaxation cassette by reciting the instructions into a tape recorder. If you have a friend or relative with a melodious voice, ask for help in making the tape. The pace should be slow and gentle, with pauses of five to ten seconds between suggestions.

Do this exercise in a room with dim lights and quiet privacy. Loosen your clothing and lie down flat or with a small pillow. Spend a few minutes on a deep breathing pattern. Although you won't be counting, try to maintain the deep breathing throughout the exercise.

- Let your heels sink down and relax. Relax your feet. Your calves feel soft and relaxed. Relax your thighs. Your legs feel long and relaxed.
- Breathe deeply into your abdomen. As you exhale, let your buttocks soften and relax. Let your lower back melt. Feel the relaxation flowing up your spine. Your middle back feels very lengthened and relaxed. Your rib cage feels expanded and relaxed. Your shoulder blades feel open and relaxed. Your chest is expanded and relaxed. Your breathing is deep and effortless.
- Relax your fingers. Feel the relaxation flowing up your arms. Your arms feel long and relaxed. The relaxation flows into your shoulders. Let the tops of your shoulders soften.
- The relaxation flows from your arms up the sides of your neck, up your spine, and up the back of your neck. Your neck feels long and soft. Your throat feels calm. Let your head sink into the floor. You don't have to hold anything up. Just let go. Let your jaw and your mouth soften. Relax your face and your eyes. Your forehead feels very smooth.
- Your entire body from your toes to your head is completely relaxed. You inhale peace and good health with every breath. You don't have to be anywhere or do anything but relax. It is safe to let go completely. Melt into total relaxation.

> Spend a few minutes enjoying the blissful serenity. This peaceful state is your true self, your inner self, and it's always there waiting for you.

When you feel ready, stretch your body gently, as if you're just waking up, rejuvenated and filled with a sense of well-being. Try to keep this feeling with you throughout the day.

At first, you may find that this exercise puts you to sleep. When you let go of muscular tension your body might naturally fall into a state of restorative sleep. Perhaps you'll wake up without a headache. Some people who have trouble sleeping find it a wonderful way to cure insomnia. Eventually, however, you will learn that you can be totally relaxed and fully awake. You will experience the joy of conscious relaxation.

Meditation

For thousands of years people have used meditation as a way to quiet, focus, and develop their minds. During the last two decades, a great deal of attention has been paid to the benefits of meditation in stress reduction. Hundreds of scientific studies and articles attest to the physiological changes that individuals undergo when they meditate.

There are many excellent forms of meditation, primarily yogic and Zen practices. These methods can be highly beneficial both in reducing the health hazards of stress and in expanding your consciousness.

One of the most popular forms of meditation is Transcendental Meditation (TM), introduced to the Western world by Maharishi Mahesh Yogi. This system involves the repetition of a mantra, a specific sound for the mind to focus on. TM proponents insist that the mantra is a highly personal secret and must be assigned by a special teacher during a costly ritual.

There is no doubt that TM is highly beneficial in reducing stress; this is well-documented in research studies. There is quite a bit of dispute, however, about whether a secret mantra is necessary.

Many meditators experience the benefits of mantra meditation with a word they choose themselves. The Sanskrit word "Om" is called the universal mantra and is a wonderful meditation tool. If you are not comfortable with this mantra, you might try the word "one."

To practice mantra meditation, sit up straight with your hands in your lap in a quiet room. Close your eyes and focus on deep breathing. Repeat your mantra on every exhalation. It can be repeated silently or softly vocalized. When other thoughts or images come into your head, allow them to pass and keep focusing on the mantra. This meditation can be practiced ten to twenty minutes at a time, one to three times a day. When you are finished meditating, remain seated quietly for a few minutes before getting up.

Meditation is simple, but not always easy. It usually takes some practice before you can completely focus your thoughts on the meditation. Paradoxically, the key to success is not trying too hard. Don't try to push the thoughts out of your head; just let them float out and return your mind to the meditation. Don't attempt to fight the intruding thoughts; simply let them go. Maintain a passive and relaxed attitude. If your concentration wavers, don't get angry or frustrated. Relaxation training is about learning to be kind and gentle with yourself.

A Guided Relaxation

Some of our headache patients find it difficult to concentrate when they try doing relaxation exercises or meditating on their own. In response to their needs, we created a special guided relaxation cassette tape with soothing background music.

You can order this tape by contacting our office (see p. 178 for address). Or you can make your own personalized cassette by using the text, which we have included here. You can record it in silence or with a favorite piece of serene music playing softly in the background. It should run about twenty minutes and be paced so that the listener can assimilate all the suggestions.

/ Dr. Stromfeld's Guided Relaxation /

Lie on your back and get into a comfortable position. Allow your eyes to close and become aware of your breathing. Breathe deep into your abdomen and feel your belly rise with oxygen as you breathe in. Become aware of your body position and the way you tend to hold your body. Allow your body to relax and let go.

Imagine your body is like a balloon and that this balloon is your favorite color. When you breathe in allow the balloon to fill with oxygen; when you breathe out let the balloon in your body collapse and let go. Allow your body to become soft. The floor is strong. You can let go. You've held on for your whole life and your body has responded to that. Now is the time to let it go.

Imagine floating on a cloud. Continue to breathe in and out, and with each breath, allow your body to fill up with oxygen. When you let it out relax your body. With each breath, relax more and more.

Imagine five holes on the bottom of each foot and in the palms of each hand. When you breathe in, feel the oxygen and air come up through the holes in your feet and palms, travel up your limbs, and fill your abdo-

men. As it does this, all the muscles relax and let go. With every breath you take, you bring a source of energy into your body. Oxygen is a tremendous source of energy. It is all around us and in us. It nourishes us and allows us to be healthy. Breathe in and allow the oxygen to come up through the holes in your feet.

At the same time, feel the breath going through your nose and head and upper part of your body, nourishing and relaxing. With every breath you take, you bring a source of energy to every part of your body. At the same time that it energizes you, it also relaxes you. Every gland, organ, muscle, and cell of your body is relaxed and energized, nourished by this oxygen that is all around us. See this oxygen as white light. This light heals your body. It energizes every system of your body and refocuses your body's self-healing mechanism.

The body has its own computer system; what we're going to do now is turn that computer system back on. So go up into your mind and see a switch that says "Computer On," and gently flip it. The switch is now activating the computer of your body. Now turn on all the lights in your body. Feel the energy surging through your entire body. And as it does so, feel the soothing, healing energy that is bringing your body up to a level of functioning that feels beautiful.

See a beam of soft, nourishing light coming down from above and surrounding your entire body with the soft white light. It is creating a cushion of light that protects and energizes your body. Allow this light to enter inside you and create a glow on the inside. Turn that glow up so that it fills you from head to toe. Now let this glow surround the outside of your body. This light heals you and protects you. It is a cushion that allows only good things in and keeps all bad things out. With every breath you take you reenergize the source of white light. You are protected now.

Every time you listen to this tape you will become more relaxed and more energized; centered. You are nourishing your body and soul. You can regain this sense of freedom, energy, and peace at any time by simply becoming aware of your breathing. A few times every day, become aware of your breathing for thirty seconds and breathe deep into your abdomen to recapture this feeling. Breathe at any time of the day when you are feeling stress. With each breath your body will relax and you will become more in control of the situation and of your life.

You are a special person, the likes of which this world will never see again. Enjoy each day. Live in the moment. The past is but a memory, and the future is a hope and a dream. Life is to be lived one moment at a time. In every moment you can have a moment of peace.

See the word "love" or the words "I love you" and bring them into your body. See the words travel throughout your entire body, touching every part. Feel the sensation that it creates.

At the count of three, bring yourself back to this room, fully awake, full of energy, and ready to meet the world, ready to create a beautiful day. One, two, three. Open your eyes, fully refreshed, with a sense of wholeness. And have a beautiful day. You can create it because you are a special person.

Creative Imagery

The guided relaxation we've just done makes use of creative imagery, or visualization. Creative imagery has the opposite effect of worry and negative thinking. It is a way of using your mind to create a positive, healing state. Many people believe in the power of prayer and positive thinking. Creative imagery is another form of these same impulses. It is a method of reaching and influencing your subconscious and your higher self, a way to direct your deep thoughts to create well-being instead of tension and headaches. Creative imagery helps you feel in charge of your own destiny.

It's best to do your imagery practice after a relaxation exercise, when you are at your most open and receptive. You can do any of the exercises given above to achieve this conducive state.

We will present several visualizations that are specifically geared toward helping headaches. Focus on only *one* visualization at each session; try another one the next day. When you find an image that is particularly successful, continue to use it.

The following creative imagery techniques can be used while you are experiencing a headache:

- As you breathe in, imagine that you are filling yourself with white light. The light is saturating your bones, tissues, muscles, blood vessels. It is very healing and soothing. It is filling up your head. There is no room for pain in your head as the white light fills it. Your head is free of pain and filled with blissful white light. (You can do this same visualization with blue, orange, or golden healing light.)
- Imagine that with every breath you are inhaling a magical elixir that eases the pain in your head. With every exhalation you are exhaling the pain. Keep inhaling the elixir and exhaling the pain until it is all gone.
- Imagine that you are in a very peaceful and beautiful place: a beach or the countryside. See, smell, and hear this retreat, a place where you have no pressures, no worries, no pain. Imagine a cool stream of water washing away your headache.

- Ask your headache what it is trying to tell you. Is there something you should or shouldn't be doing? Once the pain has told you what to do, it can go away. Imagine it flowing out of your head. Picture yourself in perfect good health, surrounded by golden glowing light.
- Visualize a sphere of light that starts as a pinprick and then grows to the size of a ball. Then picture the sphere getting smaller, shrinking until it disappears. Now you are going to do the same thing with the head pain. Picture it growing, expanding. Then it starts shrinking. It gets smaller and smaller until it is only a pinprick of pain. Then it disappears. (In addition to using creative imagery during a headache to reduce pain, you can use it as a preventive technique.)
- Visualize yourself experiencing a stressful situation at work. Instead of developing a headache, you react by asserting your needs, acting in a strong and effective manner, or taking a relaxing break.
- Imagine that you feel a migraine coming on. Instead of panicking, you do some self-massage and relaxation techniques. The migraine attack never begins; you feel well and relaxed.
- Visualize yourself resisting a craving for a food that causes allergic headaches. You eat something healthy instead. You enjoy the healthy food and feel satisfied.

Although imagery is most powerful if you do it directly after relaxation, once you become familiar with this technique you can "take it on the road." You can use imagery anywhere, any time you feel the need. The possibilities of this technique go far beyond helping headaches. Creative visualization can be used to help you work through almost any problem. You can become the architect of your own life! Many of the things you imagine will become a part of your reality.

Affirmations

Affirmations—positive statements that penetrate to the subconscious—can work hand in hand with creative imagery to help you use the power of your mind to create health and happiness in your life. Sometimes we are sabotaged by negative thoughts and beliefs that we hold in our subconscious minds. Affirmations work to change these negative ideas into positive ones. They are always stated simply and in the present tense to "affirm" that the statements are true, even if they are not yet manifested in reality.

You can do affirmations any time, but the optimal time is when you are relaxed: after doing a relaxation technique, in the morning directly after waking, before falling asleep, or after a bath or other relaxing activity. At these times, your mind is at its most receptive.

Affirmations can be said out loud or repeated silently to yourself, chanted, whispered, or sung. Writing them down repetitively is a powerful technique. You can also write down your affirmations and paste them up in different places: a desk drawer, a bedside table, a car dashboard. Many people find it helpful to put their written affirmations on the bathroom mirrors, so they focus on them first thing in the morning. Choose two or three affirmations to concentrate on for a week or two. Then you can try some different ones.

You can make up your own affirmations about anything: Just remember to state them in a simple, positive manner, in the present tense. Here are some examples of affirmations you might find helpful:

I deserve to feel healthy and well.
I have faith in my ability to eliminate headaches.
I can prevent headaches.
I am free of pain.
I am in perfect good health.
I live a healthy, pain-free life.
I am relaxed and confident at work.
I am confident and calm when I face challenges.
My relationships are peaceful and happy.
I express all my needs to my loved ones.
I eat only healthy, natural food that makes me feel well.
My body feels balanced and well.
I am good to my body, and it is good to me.
I am filled with inner peace and well-being.
I love myself.
I totally accept myself.

Now, you may be thinking, "Why should I say those things when they're not true?" The reason is that affirmations have an amazing capacity to come true once you start believing them. Repetition helps you believe them on a deep level and program your subconscious in a positive direction that promotes good health. Try to let go of your cynicism and give affirmations a chance. You may be very pleasantly surprised at the results.

Psychotherapy

Many people find that dealing with their emotional issues through psychotherapy helps alleviate their headaches. Once they are able to talk about their anger, guilt, fear, or anxiety, the physical ailments that these emotions can lead to no longer plague them. It is not always necessary to find answers to one's problems;

sometimes simply airing them helps both physically and psychologically.

You may be discouraged from seeking psychological help if you think it means spending twenty years on a couch talking about your childhood. Be assured that there are now a wide variety of alternatives in the mental health care marketplace. Therapy need not be an extremely long-term or expensive proposition.

There is a new breed of psychotherapists who use a holistic approach. These modern psychotherapists use a variety of therapeutic techniques from different schools of thought. Some of them use relaxation techniques, creative visualizations, bodywork, and nutritional counseling in addition to behavioral modification. In some cases, the results are quick and dramatic.

Gestalt therapy is a growth-oriented system of psychotherapy that emphasizes the here and now. Clients are encouraged to pay attention to three zones of awareness: the inner zone, where the bodily sensations and emotions are experienced; the middle zone, where thoughts, fantasies, and analyses dwell; and the outer zone, where the world is contacted through the five senses. By paying careful attention to all these levels, the "Gestalt," which means the "whole picture," emerges.

Janet Damon, a New York City psychotherapist, uses the following Gestalt technique with some of her clients who suffer from headaches: She hands them a pillow and tells them to act out on the pillow what the headache feels like. They might bang, twist, hammer, drill, or poke their fingers into the pillow. At the same time, she suggests that they make a nonverbal sound that expresses the way they feel inside their heads. They might scream, grunt, groan, whatever feels right.

"I tell them to give the headache to the pillow," says Ms. Damon. "This can be a wonderful release and a way to transfer the headache to an inanimate object.

It can also bring out the emotions behind the headache, the thoughts and feelings that were previously repressed. For this reason, it's best to do this technique with a trained therapist who can help you deal with the emotions that arise."

Another Gestalt technique is to ask clients to go inside their heads and experience their headaches as fully as possible. During this exercise images that can aid in understanding the reasons behind the headaches may emerge. Often, simply experiencing the pain as opposed to fighting it can alleviate the headache.

Cognitive therapy, which is being used by more and more mental health professionals, differs greatly from traditional psychoanalysis. Cognitive therapy is a practical approach that often yields rapid results. The basic premise is that your moods and feelings are based on your thoughts, or cognitions, and the way you interpret and perceive matters. Your inner dialogue creates your emotional responses. Depression and anxiety are caused by negative, illogical, distorted thoughts. Therefore, if you change the way you think and speak to yourself, your mood will change, and your health may improve.

Cognitive therapists help their clients gain a better understanding of their thought processes and how these affect their moods. Through dialogue with their therapists and through written exercises, clients learn to identify distortions in their thought patterns, and to adopt more rational ways of thinking that build, rather than erode, self-esteem.

For example, you might think: "I'm always making mistakes at my job." This negative thought might make you anxious at work and lead to frequent tension headaches. The cognitive distortion involved in this statement is that it is an overgeneralization and a magnification of your faults. The word "always" is an unrealistic one to use in this context. A more rational statement would be: "Sometimes I make mistakes at my job; most people do. Usually I do quite well at my job and I take pride in my work." If you can begin to think in this more positive way, you may be less anxious at work and less likely to develop tension headaches.

Somato Emotional Release

Somato emotional release was recently developed by Dr. John Upledger, a prominent osteopath and scientific researcher. He discovered that emotional tension often creates distortions in the physical structure of the human body. This can lead to changes in the tension of the connective tissue (fascia) within the body, as well as negative changes in the functioning of the muscles, spine, nervous system, circulatory, digestive, and endocrine systems. Dr. Upledger developed a treatment program that is now being used by many chiropractors, osteopaths, physical therapists, and other bodyworkers.

When health professionals use somato emotional release, they literally unwind the body, using gentle and effective techniques. While they do this work, they ask their patients to stay in touch with the emotions that arise. Often patients remember emotional traumas that were previously repressed and locked away in both their minds and bodies. This technique can free patients from the adverse effects of these hidden and often forgotten traumas.

Neuro-Linguistic Programming

Neuro-Linguistic Programming, or NLP, was developed by John Grinder, a prominent linguist, and Richard Bandler, a Gestalt therapist, mathematician, and computer wizard. They combined their talents to study how communication—both with others and within our own minds—affects our nervous system. NLP is the study of how we think and how our minds work. NLP teaches people to use their minds and communicative skills to help change their lives and achieve optimum results in whatever they choose to do.

One of the basic premises of NLP is that we have two choices: We can let our minds run us or we can take more control over them. It has been said that we use only 5 to 10 percent of the capabilities of our minds. NLP practitioners train people to gain access to a larger proportion of their minds, enabling them to create physiological changes in their body.

The following NLP procedure is a simple one that you can do yourself when you have a headache:

Lie down and close your eyes. Imagine a cloud above your head. Imagine that the headache pain is in the form of smoke. With each exhalation, breathe the smoke/pain into the cloud, until the cloud turns into an ugly, scary picture. Change this picture into a pleasant, soft, gentle scene, such as a field of grass and flowers or a placid lake. As you inhale, breathe this pleasant picture back into your head. You should feel an immediate reduction in the level of pain associated with the headache.

NLP can be a remarkable therapeutic tool. Steven Goldstone, a trainer and master practitioner at the New York Training Institute for Neuro-Linguistic Programming, endured a bout of migraine headaches a few years ago.

"I had never had headaches before, but all of a sudden I started getting one every two or three weeks. This went on for six months," said Mr. Goldstone. "I explored many possible physical causes, but I found no answers and the migraines continued."

Mr. Goldstone used an NLP process called reframing to get in touch with his unconscious mind. He discovered that the migraines were a message from his unconscious mind to make him aware that he was thinking negatively about a personal aspect of his life, and that it was important to change these negative thoughts and beliefs into positive, constructive ideas. Once he did this, he stopped getting migraines. Now Mr. Goldstone uses reframing and other NLP techniques to help some of his clients who suffer from headaches.

Hypnosis

Hypnosis can be used as a separate therapy, or in conjunction with other modalities, such as NLP or psychotherapy. Hypnotists may give direct suggestions regarding headaches. The success of this approach varies widely according to the quality of the hypnotist and the receptivity of the subject. More often, hypnosis is used in an indirect way to deal with headaches. The hypnotist helps the subject get in contact with the unconscious emotions contributing to headaches. Hypnosis can also help people learn to relax different parts of the body and to increase blood circulation, which can be effective in some cases.

Delving Deeper

Some of the mind/body techniques we have been describing may sound too mystical or strange for you. Although these techniques have proven helpful for many headache sufferers, they require a certain frame of mind in order to be optimally effective. If you have no faith in a method and feel certain that it wouldn't help you, it probably won't.

One of the best ways to develop faith in your ability

to control and improve your mind/body is to learn more about these techniques. Some, particularly meditation, creative imagery, psychotherapy, and NLP, may require further study in order for you to reach a complete understanding. If any of these topics intrigue you, why not learn more about them? The more you learn, the more expansive and healthy your life can be. You can check the "Suggested Further Reading" section in the back of this book, or visit a bookstore or library and find your own sources.

Biofeedback

We hope you will be open-minded enough to try different mind/body techniques with a positive attitude. However, if you can't overcome your skepticism, or if these approaches don't work for you, you might want to try a method that is indisputably modern and scientific: biofeedback.

Biofeedback means bringing information and awareness of biological functions into the conscious mind. Biofeedback training involves the measurement of physiological functions so that the individual can learn to exert control over them. Biofeedback training can teach people how to control muscle tension and blood flow.

Many research studies have been done to document the success of biofeedback training in helping patients with both tension and migraine headaches. The statistics vary, but a general estimate is that 50 to 70 percent of those who receive biofeedback training experience some benefit. Some people learn to prevent headaches, others manage to reduce the intensity and duration of the pain.

Richard C., a structural engineer, had frequent tension headaches for most of his adult life. "I knew stress was involved, but I couldn't see myself getting into meditation or one of those way-out things. Not my style. But biofeedback training seemed substantial and scientific. So I decided to give it a try."

Richard went to a biofeedback training center. The therapist asked him to fill out a detailed questionnaire about his health history, the nature of his pain, and his personal habits. He was asked to keep a pain diary for two weeks, charting the frequency and quality of his headaches. "I got kind of impatient at this point; I was hoping for some fast action. But I did as I was told," said Richard.

When Richard returned for his second visit, he was taken into a dimly lit, quiet room and asked to sit in a comfortable chair. The therapist showed him the biofeedback equipment and explained how it worked. "I found this reassuring," said Richard. "I trust machines."

The first type of biofeedback training Richard received was electromyographic (EMG) feedback, which is most frequently used to help tension headaches. After his face was cleansed with alcohol, three electrodes were placed on his forehead. He was asked to relax. A measurement was taken of the electrical force generated by the muscle tension in his forehead; this was a threshold measurement. The therapist then set the machine to produce a soft tone to correspond to this measurement. Richard was asked to try to relax his forehead muscles even more. When he succeeded in doing this, the sound ceased. The tone was then set at a lower threshold, and he was asked to relax further until that tone was also terminated.

In subsequent EMG feedback sessions, the electrodes were placed on his jaw, cheeks, temples, neck, and shoulders, and around his ears to measure the different muscles involved in headaches. Gradually, Richard learned to lower his resting muscle tension level to a point where it could no longer cause headaches. "There was a nice side benefit. A crick in my neck stopped bothering me."

Richard also learned to combat the stress response through finger temperature, or thermal feedback. The temperature in his finger was measured as an indication of the blood flow to the hand. Richard learned to increase the blood flow and raise the temperature. This has a similar effect as the autogenic training technique during which you think of being "warm and heavy."

Although you can buy biofeedback machines to use at home, it is not practical to walk around with electrodes attached to your head or fingers. One of the goals of biofeedback training is to learn to experience biofeedback awareness without the machines. Once Richard had learned to reduce his muscle tension and increase his blood flow with the monitoring of the machines, he embarked on the voluntary control phase of his training.

During the voluntary control phase, the therapist monitored his progress, but Richard was now shown the results. He learned to experience relaxation without the machines feeding him information. He was also encouraged to practice the control techniques at home.

"The machines showed me the concrete evidence I needed to see. They helped me learn what it feels like to truly relax. Now I'm a believer," said Richard. "When I feel my body tensing up, I take a few minutes out to physically relax. It spares me a whole lot of headaches."

Chapter Eight

Exercises to Help Headaches

By this point, you are well aware that headaches are not "all in your head," either literally or figuratively. You know that tension, nutritional deficits, and misalignments or malfunction in different parts of your body can lead to head pain. To prevent headaches you must keep your entire structure in a relaxed and balanced state. Two ways you can help do this are through maintaining proper posture and doing therapeutic exercises.

Posture

Douglas B., the editor of a corporate newsletter, spent many hours each day at his word processor. He slouched in his chair, his neck craning forward, as he studied the words on the screen. Sometimes he held the telephone between his ear and his shoulder and typed notes onto the keyboard. He blamed his frequent tension headaches on deadline pressure rather than the true cause: postural habits that caused overcontraction of his neck muscles and irritation and pinching of the nerves in his neck.

Many people exacerbate or even create their head-

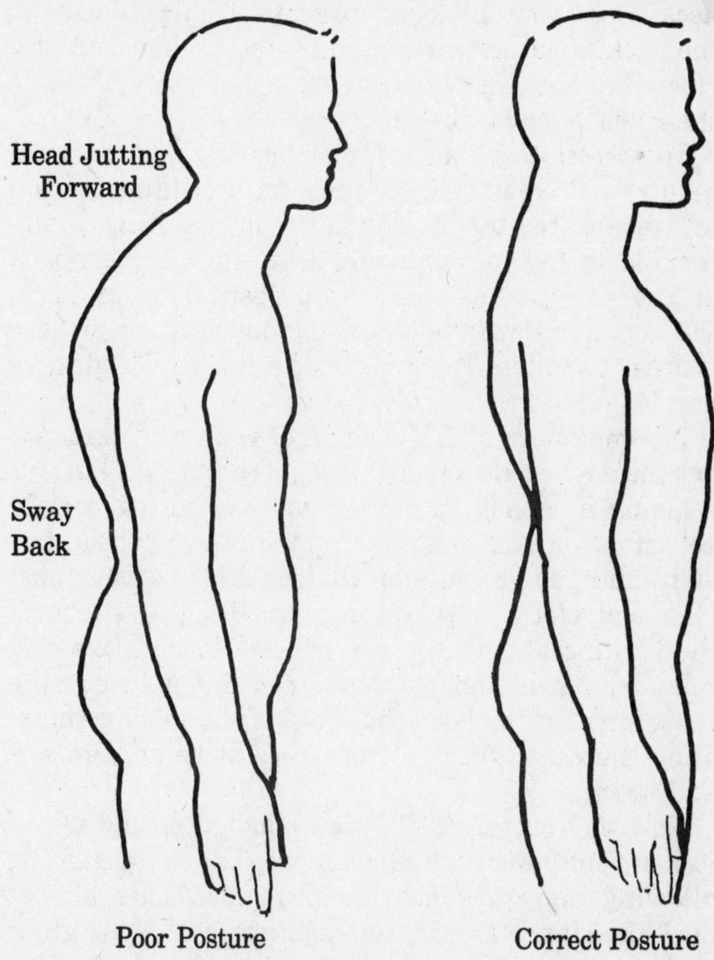

ache problems because they have poor postural habits. Indeed, poor posture is the norm; correct posture is a rarity. But with a little self-awareness and practice, you can habitually maintain a posture that reduces the amount of stress on your body.

The easiest way to check your posture is to have a friend take a side view photograph of you wearing a leotard or minimal clothing. The first point to check—

mportant for headache sufferers—is the r neck jut forward? A slight curve of ral; it should not be ramrod straight. many people develop a habit of thrusting heads too far forward.

To correct this habit, remember the balloon technique in Chapter Three: Imagine a helium balloon attached to the top of your head, pulling it up. Imagine, too, lifting your chin and drawing your head back at the point where your skull rests on your neck. When you're trying to lengthen your neck, make sure it doesn't tighten. Try to develop a feeling of lightness and length.

Become aware of the position of your neck throughout the day: when you are eating, reading, working, or relaxing at home. In all probability, during certain activities you are most likely to crane your head forward and put pressure on the sensitive nerves, muscles, and blood vessels. Once you become aware of these vulnerable times, you can try to lengthen and relax your neck during them. You might invoke the sense memory of how your neck feels during relaxation exercises. Think of your neck as being very soft and warm.

Now, go back to the side view photograph and take a look at your lower back. Does it sway backward slightly, allowing your abdomen to protrude? This almost ducklike stance is very common and can cause great problems. Swayback posture puts tremendous pressure on your lower vertebrae and can have a ripple effect that goes all the way up to your neck, causing constriction and head pain.

To correct swayback, think of tucking your pelvis under slightly. Do not tighten your lower back; simply let your lower vertebrae drop so they are no longer arched. Your hips should lie in the same plane as your waist instead of tilting backward. Think of pulling up like ballet dancers, whose tall, straight alignment enables them to turn and balance.

High heels are the enemy of good posture and encourage hypertension of the lower back. Try lower-heeled footware whenever possible. Remember, if you cultivate a healthy posture, you will naturally look taller and no longer need the extra inches from heels.

Now take a front view of yourself in the mirror. Is your weight shifted onto one hip or the other? If your body is aligned, your weight should be centered evenly. Many people, unfortunately, develop the habit of dropping their weight to one leg. You can correct this habit simply by pulling up through your spine. Imagine that the helium balloon floating above your head is lifting up not only your neck but your entire body.

Are your shoulders slightly hunched up or rolling forward? This causes overcontraction of the trapezius muscles and irritation to the nerves. Try to be conscious of tension and let your shoulders relax. Is one shoulder higher than the other or is one side more muscularly developed? This could be due to uneven distribution of the weight you carry.

Like many women, Susan G. carried a very large and overfilled shoulder bag. "Sometimes it seemed like I was carrying my whole closet around," she said. "Clothes for the gym, clothes to wear the next day if I was staying overnight with my boyfriend, a book, makeup, wallet, papers from work . . ." Susan was in the habit of holding her shoulder bag on her right side. This resulted in chronic tension in her trapezius muscles on the right side and a misalignment of her spinal vertebrae. Headaches were the end result of this seemingly benign habit.

Susan went to the chiropractor's office because her shoulder hurt. She was surprised to discover that this pain was connected to her headaches. After a series of chiropractic adjustments, the structural problems were cleared up, but in order to prevent them from recurring, Susan had to change her carrying habits. "It's funny how you never think of the simplest things," said Susan. "I never thought a shoulder bag could cause a headache. But now that I don't carry as much, I hardly ever get headaches."

Continually holding a large handbag or shoulder bag on one side can result in imbalance in the shoulder muscles. If you sling the strap of your bag over the opposite shoulder, the weight is more evenly distributed. You might also carry your bag cradled in your arms in front of your body. Consider using a bag of a lightweight synthetic material instead of leather, or carrying a small backpack.

Try to follow Susan's example and pare your daily load down to the bare essentials. Susan began leaving her workout clothes in the office and some spare outfits at her boyfriend's apartment. If you *must* carry a great deal, divide the load into two bags so the weight is evenly distributed to both arms.

If you carry a briefcase, try to alternate which hand you carry it in. When you are carrying groceries, divide the load into two bags instead of putting the burden all on one side. Whatever you carry or lift, try to balance the weight on both sides of your body to avoid undue strain.

Sometimes it is beneficial to get professional help with your posture. Chiropractors, osteopaths, physical therapists, exercise physiologists, fitness trainers, and yoga teachers can work on your alignment. The Alexander technique offers individualized lessons in posture and balancing body mechanics. This technique focuses on the alignment of the head, spine, and torso. Practitioners use guided imagery and gentle manual adjustment to help their clients "unlearn" lifelong bad habits.

The Feldenkrais method reeducates the body to create better alignment, range of motion, and coordination. This method has two major components: Functional Integration, during which practitioners gently manipulate their clients' bodies so that they gain insight into how they move; and Awareness Through Movement, a series of exercises.

Practitioners of both the Alexander technique and the Feldenkrais method can be found in most major cities. There are also books for self-instruction on these teachings.

Preventive Exercises

When tension accumulates in your body, it can lead to overcontracted muscles and headaches. Gentle stretching exercises can help release tension and maintain alignment. Here is a simple routine that can help prevent headaches. Although it begins with an overall body warm-up, this routine focuses on stretching the neck and shoulders, the parts of the body most often involved in head pain.

You may decide to do the routine when you wake up, in order to dispel the stiffness of sleep and begin the day with a stretched and relaxed body. You can also do this series during the day, to alleviate the tension that accumulates during work. A stretching break is much more beneficial than a coffee break, especially if you are prone to headaches. You might also do the routine after work in order to disperse the muscle tension that builds up by the end of the day.

Upper Body Stretching Routine

1. Begin by standing up, with your feet about six inches apart. Concentrate on centering your body and lifting into an aligned posture. Breathe

slowly and feel the breath travel throughout your body.

2. Lift your right arm and stretch it above your head, lengthening the entire right side of your body. Then let your right arm float gently down to your side. Lift your left arm and stretch it above your head, lengthening the entire left side of your body. Then let your left arm float down to your side. Repeat this stretch on the right side and on the left side. Then lift both arms overhead and stretch your entire body. Exhale and let your arms float down.
3. Drop your head to your chest. Roll your spine down toward the floor slowly, one vertebra at a time. Bend your knees slightly as you roll down. Don't overstretch; just go as far as you can comfortably. Your hands might touch the floor, or they might be many inches from the ground, depending on your level of flexibility. Maintain the position for about five seconds, relaxing and letting the weight of your head stretch you out. Then bend your knees deeper and begin to roll up slowly from the bottom of your spine, one vertebra at a time, holding your stomach in, with your head coming up last.

   When you reach a fully erect posture, stretch your right arm up to the side and reach overhead toward your left side. Bring your right arm back and down as you center your body. Stretch your left arm up to the side and reach overhead toward your right side. Bring your left arm back and down as you center your body. Take a deep breath, then do this entire sequence once again.
4. Now that your body is warmed up, you are ready to stretch your neck and shoulders. Slowly drop your head to your chest. Lift your head center.

Arch your head back very slightly. Think of lifting your head up and only slightly back, rather than dropping it down. Feel a gentle stretch in the front of your neck. Hold this position for five seconds and then return your head to center.*

5. Turn your head to the right and hold for five seconds, then return to center. Turn your head to the left and hold for five seconds, then return to center.
6. Drop your right ear toward your right shoulder. Place your right hand on your left shoulder to prevent it from rising up. Hold for five seconds, then lift your head to center. Drop your left ear toward your left shoulder. Place your left hand on your right shoulder and hold for five seconds. Then lift to your head to center.
7. Begin by dropping your head to your chest. Slowly circle your head to the right three times. You can let your head drop completely to the front and the sides, but keep it slightly lifted to the back. Think of making an egg or oval shape with your head, rather than a complete circle. After three ovals to the right, rotate your head to the left three times, then lift to center.
8. Lift both shoulders up toward your ears, then let them drop gently. Do this five times. Keeping your shoulders down, press them toward your back, then move them center, then squeeze them together toward the front. Do this five times in each direction.

*Never let your head drop all the way back while doing this exercise or any other arching movements, as this puts too much pressure on your neck. The head movement to the back is very small and controlled. You can tell that you are arching too far if the skin at the back of your neck is folded. It should remain smooth. Think of lifting your head primarily *up* and lengthening it.

9. Rotate your shoulders front, up, back, and down, making a complete circle. Take your time and make the circle as wide as you can. Do this five times toward the front, then switch directions, circling back, up, and front five times.
10. Place your hands on your shoulders and circle your elbows. Touch them in front, circle up, back, and down five times, then switch direction and do five more circles.
11. Clasp your hands behind your back. Try to straighten your arms, keeping your shoulders down. Take a few deep breaths in this position and then release your hands.
12. With your arms at your sides, roll down your spine slowly, bending your knees slightly. Hang down for three seconds. Bend a little deeper, then roll up slowly, feeling tall, lifted, and aligned. Try to maintain this feeling throughout the day.

This routine may sound a bit complicated on first reading, but be assured it becomes simpler after you've done it a few times. It takes only about ten to fifteen minutes, but it can make a tremendous difference in the way you feel. You can also do bits and pieces of this routine if you don't have time to do all of it. When you feel the tension building up, take a minute to stretch where you need it most. A quick stretch may nip a headache in the bud.

Yoga

Yoga is the ultimate holistic fitness system. Yoga routines create physical and mental flexibility and strength. Both the physical limits of the body and the horizons of the mind expand through yoga.

The most widely practiced of the many branches of

yoga is hatha-yoga. The goal of hatha-yoga is to reach a state of unity with a higher consciousness through physical and mental control. Hatha-yoga practice involves breathing exercises to gain control over the breath, meditation to still the mind so that it may perceive the infinite, and postures that create a state of optimal flexibility and good health.

There are thousands of variations of the hatha-yoga postures, which are called *asanas*. Some are very simple; others take many years to achieve. While doing the postures, the practitioner tries to retain breath control and a relaxed, meditative frame of mind. This mental concentration unites the body and mind.

Those who practice yoga postures reap both internal and external benefits. A firm, toned, youthful, and flexible body are the outward results of diligent yoga practice, which can also have a tremendously positive effect on the organs, glands, and circulation. Yoga can correct many of the underlying causes of head pain, and many people have found that taking up this practice relieves their chronic headaches.

Although forms of yoga have been practiced for thousands of years, there has been an upsurge in its popularity in this country during the last two decades. Yoga classes are widely available throughout the country now, through adult schools and Y's as well as the many yoga schools. There are also scores of books and audio and videotapes for self-instruction.

Aerobic Exercise

Regularity of exercise is important in preventing headaches. Exercise can stimulate endorphin production and enhance overall functioning of all the body systems. We recommend a combination of yoga or yoga-based stretches and cardiovascular work.

Vigorous exercise can help prevent headaches by

alleviating stress, tension, and depression. But in order to reap these benefits, you must approach your exercise routine with the right spirit. Don't let concerns about performance or competition dominate; allow yourself simply to play. Instead of being judgmental, concentrate on relaxing and feeling good.

When you choose an aerobic exercise, consider the hazards as well as the benefits. Jogging can create many structural problems that lead to headaches. Aerobic dancing can also result in a very high rate of injury. Why not try a gentler form of aerobic exercise, such as brisk walking, bike riding, or swimming? Swimming has been found to be especially therapeutic for headache sufferers. A word of caution: Aerobic exercise should not be done during a headache attack, but only when you are feeling normal. And if you experience a sudden headache during exercise; it is a signal to stop, sit down, do some deep breathing, and relax.

Bodybuilding and Calisthenics

Working with weights can put enormous strain on the neck and shoulder regions, which can lead to headaches. If you are a bodybuilder, be sure to warm up with gentle stretches and to cool down after a workout. While pumping weights, do not let your head tilt backward, as this creates compression in the neck. Keep your neck as long and relaxed as possible. Move from the shoulder joint rather than from the upper trapezius muscles. Work with a trainer who is concerned about safety as well as performance. And don't push yourself further than you are ready to go.

If you enjoy doing calisthenics, develop an awareness of your body while you are working out. Are you holding your neck stiffly? Are your shoulders tight? Remember, you can do the same movements without unnecessary tension, and you'll feel better for doing so.

Many people hold a great deal of tension in their necks while doing sit-ups. Remember, sit-ups are supposed to exercise your abdomen, not your neck. The least stressful way to do sit-ups is to lie on your back with your knees bent and your feet on the floor. Place your hands across your chest; right hand on left shoulder and left hand on right shoulder. Tuck your chin in and rise only halfway up. Try to keep your neck relaxed as you do so. If you still feel a great deal of tension in your neck, you might consider abandoning sit-ups for alternative abdominal exercises. "No pain, no gain," can be a dangerous fallacy. Knowledgeable, enlightened instructors can teach you how to stay fit without undue discomfort.

Chapter Nine

The Healing Touch

It's natural to rub your forehead when you have a headache. When someone you care about is in pain, the natural response is to pat or stroke them soothingly. These instinctive reactions are actually simple forms of massage. Massage can be as basic as a mother patting her crying baby or as complex as a licensed practitioner giving a therapeutic treatment. In one way or another, almost everyone has experienced the power of a healing touch.

Like most holistic techniques, massage benefits both the mind and the body. Emotionally, massage evokes feelings of being cared for and nurtured; relaxing and pleasurable, it can relieve the psychological tension that plays a part in many headaches.

Massage also has many positive physiological effects. It improves blood circulation and stimulates the production of red blood cells, which carry oxygen to all parts of the body. The combination of the direct pressure of massage and the increased blood circulation facilitates the removal of toxins and wastes, such as lactic acid, a by-product of exercising the muscles, from the body. These wastes can create aches and pains if they are not eliminated.

Massage increases circulation in the lymph system,

which absorbs wastes, excess proteins, and bacteria from between the body cells. Massage also relaxes the muscles and reduces chronic tension.

Exchanging Massages

You may be thinking, "I can't afford to pay for massages." A limited budget does not mean you can't enjoy massage, however. You can become a "massage buddy" with someone you know and experience one of the best things in life for free.

Sherilee P. is a young telephone operator who often developed tension headaches during her work shift. Her husband, John, had lower back trouble that was aggravated by his work on an assembly line. "Sometimes by the time we'd get home from work we'd both be exhausted from the pain. It was very depressing," said Sherilee.

Occasionally John asked Sherilee to rub his back to alleviate the pain. "I had the idea that if it helped him, maybe it would help me," said Sherilee. "So I said, 'You do me, I'll do you.' Sure enough, after he massaged my head, neck, and shoulders, my headache went away and I had all the more energy to help him." Sherilee and John expanded their knowledge of massage by taking a "Couples' Massage Class" at their local YMCA. "Now we can help each other out instead of just being miserable together."

Your massage buddy can be any friend or relative with whom you feel comfortable. Exchanging massages is one of the nicest things people can do for each other. Why not be the one to introduce this therapeutic activity to someone you care about? You will enrich the other person's life as well as your own.

To simplify the text, we will refer to the person

giving the massage as the "masseur," although the person may actually be a female "masseuse." In the context of this chapter "masseur" does not refer specifically to a professional, but to anyone who is giving a massage. The person receiving the massage will be referred to as the "partner."

Fundamentals of Massage

Massage is a highly portable therapy. You can apply self-massage techniques anywhere: at your desk, on a train, in a waiting room. But first let's explore the optimal setting for a classical massage.

Classical massage is best done in a warm and quiet atmosphere. An outdoor setting, such as the beach or a secluded backyard, is very renewing. If the outdoors is not a practical alternative, choose a peaceful, private room.

The best place to receive a massage is on a massage table, which you can either buy or make yourself. But if you don't want to go to the expense and bother of getting a massage table, there are other options. If your mattress is very firm, you can lie on your bed without a pillow. If it is not firm, you can put a piece of plywood under the mattress. You can cover a kitchen table with a piece of carpet or carpet padding. Or you can lie on a few blankets or a sleeping bag on the floor. Just be sure that the surface you are lying on is warm and soft enough so you feel comfortable. Cover whatever surface you use with an old sheet to absorb the massage oil. The lighting should be low and indirect. The telephone should be turned off or put in another room so there are no jolting disturbances.

Oil helps make the massage a smooth and pleasant experience. Commercial massage oils are sold in many health food stores and erotica shops, but can be costly. You can make your own massage oil by mixing ordinary safflower, coconut, or almond oil with a few drops of lemon, eucalyptus, or perfume essence. If possible, warm the oil on the stove before the massage, then transfer it to a plastic squeeze bottle or a liquid soap dispenser. The oil should be applied to the masseur's hands, rather than directly to your body.

A few minutes of deep breathing can put you in a relaxed state so that you can fully benefit from the massage. You might also do one of the body relaxation exercises you learned in Chapter Seven. During the massage itself, try not to let any anxious thoughts interfere with the experience. Allow yourself to be fully in the moment, appreciating and savoring every stroke.

Feel free to tell your masseur what feels good, where you need to be touched, or if any sharp pain arises. Otherwise, try to keep conversation to a minimum. You'll probably find that it is more natural to let out incoherent moans and murmurs than to speak any words.

Classical Massage

Classical massage is probably as old as humanity itself, but its first recorded use was in ancient Greece. The Greeks incorporated massage into their daily lives and also into their medical treatments. Socrates and Plato stated that only food was more vital to life than massage. The Romans adopted many of the Greek massage techniques and spread them throughout the world. But it was not until 1914 that classical massage was formalized into a scientific technique by Peter Ling of Sweden. It is because of Mr. Ling's influential work and the school he established that classical massage is sometimes referred to as Swedish massage.

Here are some basic rules for classical massage:

- Consult a holistic doctor before embarking on a massage program to make sure it is safe for your particular case.
- Never give a massage to a seriously sick or injured person; consult a licensed professional instead.
- Keep fingernails short and even and remove any jewelry from the hands and wrists.
- A massage should not cause sharp pain. If pain does occur, the masseur should be informed immediately and stop working on that area.

You may feel discomfort when your muscles release or sensitive points are touched during a massage. This "good" pain feels somewhat pleasurable even as it hurts; it is never sharp. Try to stay in close touch with your feelings during the massage and differentiate between benign discomfort and the more intense pain that indicates that there is too much pressure on that part of your body.

/ Classical Massage for Headache Sufferers /

There are few experiences more pleasurable and therapeutic than an overall body massage. Because of practical considerations of time and energy, however, it is not always possible to cover the whole body. When this is the case, you will want your masseur to concentrate on your head, neck, and shoulders because they are the areas most frequently involved in headaches.

If your masseur is inexperienced, ask him to study the following instructions, which detail techniques that can be used either as a preventive measure or to alleviate pain during a headache attack.

/ Instructions for the Masseur /

Your partner should lie down on his or her back. If the massage is taking place on the floor, sit cross-legged above your partner's head. If your partner is on the bed, you can sit above his or her head on the bed, if this is appropriate and comfortable. Or you can draw up a chair and have your partner place his or her head at the foot of the bed. If you are working on a massage table, stand above your partner's head. These are probably the most comfortable positions for you as the masseur, but feel free to improvise.

Remember to add a light coating of warm oil to your hands at intervals throughout the massage.

Before attempting to massage another person, try some of these techniques on yourself so you'll be able to judge how much pressure to exert. Also, communicate with your partner in order to learn whether you are exerting a comfortable amount of pressure. If your partner experiences intense, sharp pain, lighten your touch.

Warm-up

1. Place your thumbs in the middle of your partner's forehead. With your other fingers, slowly stroke from the forehead to the temples, then down the cheeks to the lips. Then reverse the stroke, bringing your fingers from the chin up over the cheeks and temples to the forehead. Do this three times in each direction. (Depending on the size of your hands, your thumbs may need to move a little to allow your other fingers to reach your partner's chin. If this is the case, let your thumbs slide out to the temples, then bring them back.)

2. Using all your fingertips, make small circular movements over the scalp.

The Forehead and Temples

1. With your fingers together, place your hand lengthwise across your partner's forehead. As you stroke down to the tip of the nose with the palm of one hand, place the other on the hairline. Continue with a hand-over-hand movement, so the forehead is always covered. Do this ten times.
2. Place your right hand in the center of the forehead with your fingertips at the top of the nose. Place your left hand over your right. Use your left hand to press down on your right. Exert steady pressure for thirty seconds.*
3. Place your hands lengthwise across your partner's forehead so the heels of your hands are over the temples. Your fingertips may overlap in the center. Press down for thirty seconds.*
4. Place all your fingertips except your thumbs at the hairline in the center of your partner's forehead. Stroke in a circular motion down to the eyebrows, across the brows to the temples and back up to the hairline. Complete five slow circles.
5. With your thumbs anchored at the center of your partner's forehead, place three fingertips on the temples. Gently circle the temples with your fingertips, five times clockwise and five times counterclockwise. If your partner is experiencing a headache, he or she may request that you do this movement longer; double the number of circles.

*These steady pressure techniques are particularly helpful if your partner is experiencing a headache at the time of the massage. It is important that you check with your partner to make sure you are exerting enough pressure to have an effect, but not so much as to cause sharp pain.

Eyes and Nose Techniques

Never massage directly on the eyes or eyelids. Instead, work on the areas around the eyes. These areas are delicate; do not exert as much pressure on them as you do on the forehead.

1. Place your thumbs on the center of the browbones at the top of the nose, one thumb on each side. Pressing upward against the browbones, and avoiding direct pressure on the eyes, stroke outward toward the temples. Complete the movement with three small circles on the temples. Then return the thumbs to the nose and do this sequence three more times.
2. Start with two fingertips, one from each hand, at the top of the nose. Stroke along the eyebrows, down the temples to the cheekbones, across the cheekbones to the nose, and up the sides of the nose to the starting point. Make five complete circles around the eye sockets.

Ear and Jaw Techniques

1. Place three fingertips at the hollows underneath your partner's earlobes. Stroke up behind the ears, then down in front of the ears. Make five complete circles around the ears. Then reverse directions, stroking up in front of the ears and down behind them five times.
2. Place your thumbs in the hollows below the earlobes. Move up behind the ears, making small circles with the thumbs. Then slide the thumbs lightly down the front of the ears. Do this sequence three times.

3. Gently pull the earlobes down. Pull the outside of the ears away from the head, very gently. Hold for ten seconds, then release.
4. Starting with three fingers at the top of the ears, stroke down the cheeks and over the jaw to the center of the chin, then back up to the ears. Do this three times.

Neck and Shoulder Techniques

1. Place your thumbs behind your partner's earlobes and your other fingers at the back of the base of the skull, just outside the cervical vertebrae. Make small circles along the hairline out toward the ears, then back to the base of the skull. Do this three times.
2. Place your hands, with your fingers pressed together, at the base of the neck. Stroke up to the hairline slowly, then back down to the base of the neck, five times.
3. Place one hand on the top of the right arm. With your fingers cupped together, stroke firmly across the shoulder and up the right side of the neck to the ear. Your partner's head will move slightly to the left as you do this. Stroke back down to the shoulder. Do this three times. Then do the same on the left side.
4. With your fingertips interlocked, place both hands under your partner's head, at the base of the skull. Press up with your fingertips, so that the head lifts slightly in an arch. Hold for ten seconds, then release.
5. Place your hands under the center of the shoulders, with your thumbs on top. Knead the tops of the shoulders between your fingertips and your thumbs.

6. Place your fingers inside your partner's armpits and your thumbs in the hollows under the collarbones, just inside the arm sockets. Massage these hollows firmly with your thumbs, using a circular movement. Then knead the area between the armpits and the hollows.

To conclude, stroke up from both shoulders to the ears. Put your thumbs behind the earlobes and your other fingertips interlocked under the head. Lengthen the neck by gently pulling the head slightly toward you. Hold for ten seconds, then release.

Massage is a highly individual matter and you may want to do variations on these techniques. Just be sure not to inflict great pain or exert too much pressure, and don't massage one place for too long.

Self-Massage

It isn't always feasible to arrange for someone else to massage you just when you need it most. But you can always be your own best friend and treat yourself to a massage. The head, neck, and shoulders are the most vital areas for headache sufferers to relax. Fortunately, they are also the areas which are easiest to massage yourself.

You can massage yourself in the morning to dispel stiffness from sleeping, after work to eliminate the tension that gathered during the day, during a headache for some soothing relief, or any other time you choose. You can even incorporate self-massage into your stretching program.

Tina D. had frequent tension headaches that disrupted her life for many years. Now she successfully utilizes self-massage and exercise to prevent headaches. "I start off massaging my neck and shoulders while I'm doing my stretching exercises, first thing in the morning. Then during the day, when I feel the tension building, I take a few moments to massage myself. At first, the people I work with looked at me like I was crazy. But when I said it helps stop headaches, they wanted to learn how."

When Tina gets home from work, she does an overall body relaxation, followed by yoga exercises. Then, before she goes to sleep, she lies on her bed flat without the pillow, and massages her shoulders, neck, and head. "People spend so much money and do all sorts of crazy things in order to feel good," said Tina. "But self-massage is legal, healthy, and cheap. Everyone should do it!"

Self-Massage Instructions

You may notice that many of the self-massage instructions are similar to the classical massage techniques you have just read. Keep in mind that these are only suggestions; you can experiment and discover new ways to massage yourself. Self-massage is most relaxing when done lying on your back, but it can also be done sitting up.

1. Begin by placing your right hand on your left shoulder. Stroke across your shoulder and up the side of your neck until your thumb is behind your ear. Rub up and down behind your ear a few times. Use your other fingertips to massage the base of your skull in a circular motion. Then stroke back down to your shoulder. Squeeze the top of your shoulder and knead it between your thumb and other fingers. Do this sequence three times. Then do this sequence three times on the

other side, using your left hand on your right shoulder.

2. Place your right thumb in the hollow under your left collarbone and your other right-hand fingers under your left armpit. Press firmly into the hollow with your thumb in a circular motion. Knead the area between the hollow and your armpit. Do this sequence on your right side using your left hand.
3. Use both hands to stroke up and down the sides of your neck three times. Feel your neck lengthen as you do this.
4. Place your thumbs behind your earlobes. Massage up and down behind your ears in a circular motion. Circle your ears with your thumbs three times in each direction.
5. Place your thumbs behind your earlobes and your intertwined fingers behind your head, at the base of your skull. Use your fingers to press your head slightly toward your chin. Hold for ten seconds, then release. Use your fingers to press your head up into a passive arch. Hold for ten seconds, then release. Let your head be completely relaxed and supported by your fingers during these movements.
6. With your thumb and your forefinger, knead up the sides of your nose.
7. Place your thumbs in the hollows between the top of your nose and your eyes. Use your thumbs to gently press upward across your eyebrows. When you reach your temples, rub them in a circular motion. Do this sequence three times.
8. Place all your fingertips except your thumbs in the center of your forehead. Stroke down your forehead, down your nose, across your cheekbones, up your temples, and back across your forehead. Make five complete circles.

9. Place your thumbs on your temples and your other fingertips in the center of your forehead. While pressing down with your thumbs, use your other fingers to rub your forehead in a circular motion.
10. If you have a headache during the self-massage, you may want to exert steady pressure on your forehead with both hands for thirty seconds.
11. Use all your fingertips to massage your scalp in small circular movements.

When you first read these instructions, they may sound a bit complicated. But when you try them, you will find that they are quite simple. You may even discover that you have already done some of these techniques instinctively.

Finger-Pressure Therapy

Finger-pressure therapy has many of the same effects as classical massage: It relaxes the muscles, improves the circulation of the vascular and lymphatic systems, and promotes dispersal and conversion of waste products. Finger-pressure therapy can relieve both the direct pain caused by muscle spasm and the referred pain that is sometimes sent along nerve pathways to other parts of the body. In some instances, headaches are due to referred pain from chronically tense muscles.

Most important, finger-pressure therapy is thought to unblock and balance the energy flow within the body, thereby restoring proper functioning in the organs, glands, and physiological systems. This is the ancient basis for Oriental finger-pressure therapies, such as shiatsu and acupressure, and it has been upheld by many modern scientific discoveries.

Traditional Oriental wisdom states that there are pathways of energy, called meridians, which travel throughout the body. The meridians supply the organs, muscles, glands, and other body parts with energy, or life force. This vital life force is called "*chi*" or "*qi*" in Chinese and "*ki*" in Japanese. When the meridians are blocked, the energy flow is disrupted, and the body part served by that meridian can malfunction, with pain or illness as a result.

In acupressure, the fingers (usually the thumbs) are used at specific points, much in the same way that acupuncture needles are, to help balance and restore the normal flow of *chi* in the energy pathways. In shiatsu, an ancient Japanese system developed from Chinese techniques, finger pressure is used to "unclog" the *tsubos* (points along the meridians). This is meant to restore proper functioning to the various body structures and systems that are served by these meridians.

Trigger-point work is a modern outgrowth of these ancient modalities. It focuses on applying pressure to trigger points: points where there is a buildup of crystallized chemical by-products that either cause pain in the area or refer pain to another part of the body. Trigger-point work can be done manually or by a holistic professional using a combination of ultrasound and electrical muscle stimulation.

When you practice finger-pressure techniques, your fingernails should be short and even and your hands and wrists free of any jewelry. There is no actual massaging done in finger-pressure therapy. Instead, steady pressure is exerted with the fingers, especially the thumbs, to specific points. The finger pressure is applied with the flat part of your fingers, not the tips.

Be careful never to gouge. And never apply pressure to a swollen or injured area.

To get an idea of how much pressure should be exerted, press your fingers on the bathroom scale until it registers about seven pounds. This is how much force should be used on your head, face, or neck. Then press on the scale until you reach about twelve pounds. You can exert this much pressure on your shoulders and back.

The self-help techniques presented here are a combination of shiatsu, trigger-point work, and acupressure. Certain specific pressure points frequently help headaches. Do some exploratory work as well: Press lightly at intervals until you find a trigger point, then press firmly. Trigger points are usually easily recognizable; they feel tender, sensitive, and often painful.

Finger-Pressure Techniques to Help Headaches

Unless specifically stated otherwise, use ten seconds of steady pressure on the points mentioned.

1. With your forefingers, press in the hollows at the top of your nose, where your nose meets your eye socket (being careful never to press on the eyes). Move your forefingers along your browbones, pressing down gently at intervals. If you hit a trigger point, exert steady pressure. With your thumbs, press on the outside corners of your eye sockets. Press your thumbs and forefingers on the outside corners of the bottom ridge of your eye sockets.
2. Press with one thumb on the center of the top of your nose. Slide your forefingers down to the outside of your nostrils, and press.

3. Press at intervals over your cheekbones, around your mouth, and over your jaw. Exert pressure on any trigger points you find.
4. Press on the center of your temples with your thumbs. Use all your fingers to explore your scalp for trigger points and exert thumb pressure on any sensitive spots you discover. Run your fingers over your forehead to search out trigger points and exert forefinger pressure on any you find.
5. Place your thumbs under your earlobes at the top of your jaw and press upward. Press up on your skull right behind your ear, exerting pressure on any trigger points you feel. At the portion of your skull right behind the top of the ear, pause to press down for ten seconds. Explore in front of your ear for any trigger points that need to be released.
6. Place your thumbs behind your earlobes and move them out along the hairline toward the back of your head. About midway to the center, you will feel a slight depression. Press your thumbs into these depressions for twenty seconds. Press spots across the base of your skull at intervals of one-quarter inch. Use your forefingers to press just above the top neck vertebra for fifteen seconds. Move your fingers down to the base of the neck, outside the vertebrae, and press for twenty seconds with your forefingers.
7. Place three fingers at the back of your shoulders. Press (with greater force than on the head) for twenty seconds. Slide your fingers about three inches down and exert steady pressure on the points inside the shoulder blades and outside the vertebrae.
8. Press with your thumbs in the middle of the front of your shoulders. Place your thumbs under your collarbone, about two inches up from the armpit, and press down firmly for fifteen seconds.

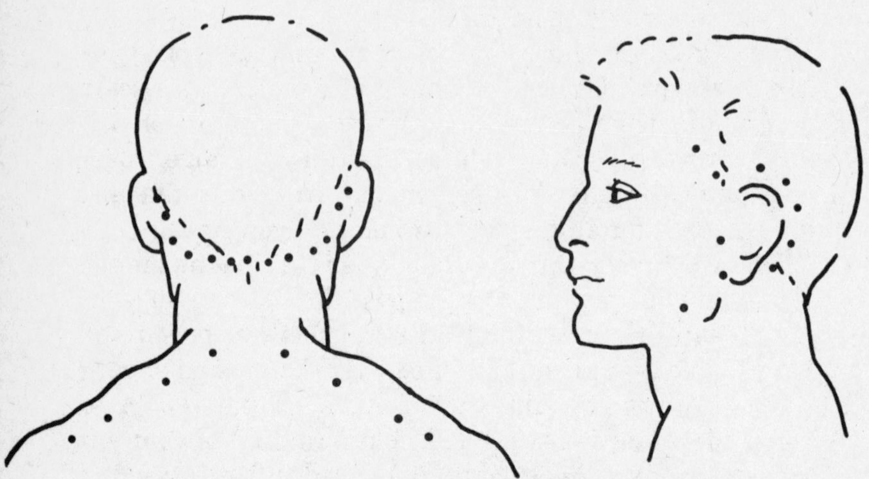

Trigger Points for Self-Massage

As you practice finger-pressure therapy, you will become familiar with where your trigger points are located and which pressure points provide the most headache relief. Then you can go directly to these points for a "quick fix" when you do not have a chance to go over your entire upper body. This can provide easy, fast, and unobtrusive pain relief when other techniques may not be appropriate.

Reflexology

Reflexology is based on the idea that all the organs, glands, and other parts of the body have corresponding reflexes on the feet. If any part of the body is malfunctioning or congested, reflexology holds that there will be tender areas in the nerve endings on the feet caused by crystalline deposits. Massaging and applying pressure to the feet will break up these deposits so that they can be carried away with other waste products. This may improve circulation and restore proper functioning to the corresponding parts of the body.

It is most relaxing if someone else gives you a reflexology treatment, but you can also do it yourself. The feet should be bare and elevated above the rest of the body. If someone else is giving you a treatment, recline and elevate your feet with pillows. If you are doing it yourself, you can cross one knee and place one leg over the other.

As with other types of massage therapy, the masseur should have short fingernails and be careful not to gouge at the feet. Usually the flat part of the thumbs are used, although the index fingers may be used as well. The technique is to press firmly and rub into each point for five to ten seconds, using up to ten pounds of finger pressure. Then you slide your finger to the next point, without losing contact with the foot. A balance should always be maintained; whatever is done to one foot should be done to the other. Work on one foot at a time.

Since headaches can be caused by malfunctions in so many different parts of the body, it's best to have a complete reflexology treatment that covers the entire foot. But the most important areas to concentrate on are the reflexes for the head, neck, and shoulders. All of these reflexes are located on the soles of the feet. These are the areas to cover:

- The big toes for the reflexes to the head
- The sides of the big toes for the reflexes to the sides of the neck

- The balls of all the other toes for the reflexes to the sinuses
- The area between the base of the second and third toes for the reflexes to the eyes
- The areas between the base of the fourth and fifth toes for the reflexes to the ears
- Under the pinky toes for the reflexes to the shoulders

Reflexology techniques can be applied to the hands as well as the feet, since the hands are also thought to have reflexes corresponding to other body parts. The hands are more convenient and accessible than the feet if you are massaging yourself.

These are the areas to cover to treat headaches:

- The bottoms of the thumbs for reflexes to the head
- The sides of the thumbs for reflexes to the sides of the neck
- The other four fingertips for reflexes to the sinuses
- Between the base of the index and middle fingers for reflexes to the eyes
- Between the base of the ring fingers and pinkies for reflexes to the ears
- Under the pinkies for reflexes to the shoulders

Hot-Compress Therapy

Bea Bonnes, a licensed massage therapist who works out of Brooklyn, New York, is a wonderful example of a holistic practitioner who helps people help themselves. She teaches her clients and a friend or relative who accompanies them how to use hot compresses to alleviate their aches and pains. "Hot compresses address the body in a focused way, zeroing in on the problem through a very gentle modality. They allow the muscles to relax at the deepest levels," says Ms. Bonnes.

It is most luxurious and therapeutic if a massage buddy does the hot-compress treatment for you, but you can also do it yourself. Use only towels that are 100 percent cotton. Each towel should be folded twice into a rectangle that is approximately nineteen inches long and four to five inches wide. They should be saturated with hot water, then wrung out. Test the water temperature by placing a towel against your cheek; it should feel very warm but not uncomfortably hot. Recline on your back with a pillow under your head and a pillow under your knees during the treatment.

For headaches caused by simple stress and muscle tension, Ms. Bonnes suggests the following procedure:

1. Place one compress behind the neck so that the towel covers the neck from ear to ear. Place another compress across the forehead, down the cheeks and over the ears. Place two compresses over the collarbone, from one shoulder point to the other. When the towels begin to cool (after about five minutes), they should be reheated under the hot water. Remove and reheat the hot compresses twice more to complete this section of the treatment.
2. For the next segment, place one towel in a doughnut shape over the face, over the forehead, eyes, ears, cheeks, and mouth and under the chin, leaving the nostrils exposed. After about five minutes, reheat this compress, then reheat it once again when it cools.

Spend a few minutes savoring the relaxation before getting up, and if you happen to fall asleep, enjoy it.

The Choice Is Yours

Some massage techniques we have discussed probably sound more appealing to you than others. One of the reasons we offer different alternatives is that everyone has a preference. One of the delightful things about massage is that there are so many choices. Try the methods that appeal most to you. You may enjoy them so much that you want to learn more.

There are many ways to study massage: instructional books and videos, courses at Y's, adult centers, massage schools, and bodywork centers, private sessions and lessons. Exploring the world of massage may add a rich new dimension to your life as well as help you conquer headaches.

Finding a Professional Massage Therapist

If you can afford the luxury, a professional massage can be extremely relaxing as well as therapeutic. One of the best ways to find a professional massage therapist is through word-of-mouth referral. Relatives, friends, colleagues, doctors, or other health professionals can be referral sources. If you wish further help in finding a massage therapist, you can contact:

Associated Professional Massage Therapists
P.O. Box 1263
3575 S. Fox
Englewood, CO 80150-1263
(303) 692-6571

This organization of bodyworkers provides referrals and public information.

Before you undergo a session with a massage therapist, we suggest that you ask certain questions, such as:

Are you licensed?

Where did you study and for how long?

How long have you been in practice?

What techniques do you use?

Do you have any methods that specifically help headaches?

May I contact any of your clients for references?

How long are your sessions and how much do they cost?

Where will the sessions take place?

Asking these questions and listening to the answers carefully will help you choose a massage therapist with whom you are comfortable. However, there is nothing like the "hands-on" experience to ensure that the massage therapist is right for you, so have a trial session before you commit to a series. Follow your instincts and continue with the massage therapist only if you feel he or she has the "right touch."

Acupuncture

Acupuncture is a five-thousand-year-old Chinese therapy that, like acupressure and shiatsu, seeks to balance and unblock the energy currents within the body. Acupuncturists believe that thin needles inserted into specific points along the meridians clear blockages and restore the energy flow (chi) to the proper balance. Many modern acupuncturists use electrical currents, heat, and/or massage in place of or in addition to the needles. These techniques have often been found to relieve pain. Some Western researchers believe that the pain-relieving effects of acupuncture are partially due to increased endorphin production.

Acupuncture can be very effective if the major cause of your headaches lies within the meridian system. Many headache sufferers do not respond to acupuncture, or experience only temporary relief, however, because the cause of their headaches lies outside the meridian system.

If you decide to explore the acupuncture alternative, it is essential that you do so with a qualified practitioner. If you would like more information about acupuncture or help in locating an acupuncturist in your area, you can call or write to:

Traditional Acupuncture Foundation
American City Building
Suite 100
Columbia, MD 21044
(301) 997-4888

CHAPTER TEN

Alternative Professional Treatments*

IN SOME CASES, SELF-HELP METHODS ARE ENOUGH TO ELIminate headaches, but many people need professional correction of the underlying causes of their pain. At the onset of your headache recovery program, you will probably need the assistance of a holistic professional to clear up imbalances that are not self-correctable. A holistic practitioner can assist you in bringing your body to a balanced and well-functioning state, so that your self-help program will be optimally effective in preventing headaches.

The health care marketplace now offers a wide variety of alternatives to traditional medicine. Instead of confusing you with a superficial explanation of *all* the holistic treatments available, we will focus on a select few. The validity of these treatments has been substantiated through extensive clinical research. These

*NOTE: This chapter covers the many and varied techniques studied by doctors of chiropractic in the seventeen chiropractic colleges in the United States.

Sadly, the state of the law in some jurisdictions has not kept pace with the state of the chiropractic arts.

The scope of practice for doctors of chiropractic varies from state to state. To determine what the scope of chiropractic is in your state you may wish to discuss the matter with your chiropractor, the state chiropractic association, or the licensing board in your state.

drug-free approaches have proven to be effective in helping many chronic headache patients lead pain-free lives.

Chiropractic Health Care

Chiropractic is a health profession that specializes in using natural approaches for correcting bodily ailments. Doctors of chiropractic are physicians who give special attention to the nervous system, musculoskeletal system, spinal biomechanics, and nutritional and environmental factors.

Since its development by Daniel David Palmer in 1895, chiropractic care has grown to be the most popular natural health care system in the Western world. Over thirty thousand chiropractors treat over ten million patients in the United States alone.

Chiropractors, also known as doctors of chiropractic or chiropractic physicians, complete between two and four years of undergraduate college, focusing on science, and then go on to complete four years at a recognized chiropractic college. Their curriculum includes the study of anatomy, physiology, chemistry, bacteriology, diagnosis, neurology, x-ray, psychology, obstetrics, gynecology, orthopedics, and nutrition, totaling approximately 4,485 class hours. In addition, chiropractic college students study manipulation, adjustment, and many other techniques, and apply their knowledge during a one-and-a-half-year internship before graduation. They must demonstrate clinical competence and pass stringent state and national examinations before they receive their licenses to practice.

Chiropractic care is based on the fact that proper functioning of the nervous system and spine are essential to good health. Misalignments, abnormal biomechanics, and imbalances of the spine can lead to a complex clinical entity called a subluxation. This can result in abnormal functioning of the nervous system, muscles, joints, and internal organs and glands, often leading to a host of bodily ailments, including headaches. To correct these imbalances, chiropractors use a variety of approaches, including hands-on techniques to manipulate and adjust the spinal vertebrae. These techniques are usually gentle and painless. They work to restore normal functioning (biomechanics) to the spine, correct the causes of irritation to the nervous system, increase the range of motion, and often correct the underlying causes of chronic pain.

While spinal manipulation and adjustments are still cornerstones of their practice, many modern, holistic chiropractors also employ other approaches to balance the body. Craniosacral therapy, TMJ work, body biomechanics (examining and correcting the functioning of the muscles and joints), neurological reeducation (specific exercises to improve the interaction between the brain, nervous system, and muscles of the body), relaxation training, nutritional counseling, and rehabilitative exercises are among the methods they may use. Postural advice and stretching and strengthening exercises for specific regions of the body are often given.

Holistic chiropractors understand that the body has innate intelligence and self-correcting mechanisms that are designed to maintain homeostasis (normal functioning of the body). Imbalances in various systems of the body interfere with homeostasis. Chiropractors often call upon therapies ranging from ancient healing methods to the most modern advances to develop balance in the minds and bodies of their patients. Once balance is reestablished, the self-correcting mechanisms can function without interference. Chiropractors also help their patients maintain balance and good health by educating them on prevention and self-care.

Imbalances in the spine, cranium (skull), TMJ, or other parts of the body structure can lead to headaches for many reasons—pinched nerves, altered function of the nervous system, hormonal disturbances, a change in the hydrostatic pressure of the cerebrospinal fluid within the cranium and central nervous system, or vascular changes in the blood vessels serving the head and neck. Since these problems are usually difficult to self-diagnose, we recommend that all headache sufferers undergo a complete chiropractic examination.

Choosing a Chiropractor

Since chiropractic is such a popular form of health care, you will probably have no trouble finding a chiropractor in your area. You can even find a list under the heading "Chiropractors" in the Yellow Pages in most regions. In addition, the American Chiropractic Association and the Motion Palpation Institute provide referrals and other information.

You can reach this association at:

The American Chiropractic Association
1701 Clarendon Boulevard
Arlington, VA 22209
(800) 368-3083

You can reach the Motion Palpation Institute at:

M.P.I.
c/o Dr. Leonard J. Faye
10780 Santa Monica Boulevard
Suite 400
Los Angeles, CA 90025
(213) 470-1225

Before selecting a chiropractor, it may help to ask the following questions to determine if the practitioner is the right one for you:

- Can you tell me about your educational background?

The practitioner should be a graduate of a fully accredited chiropractic college and be a D.C. (Doctor of Chiropractic).

- Are you a holistic chiropractor?

Although many chiropractors today are holistic, there are some who are not, meaning they do *only* spinal manipulation and adjustments, and do not address the other factors involved in achieving optimum health. While spinal adjustments are extremely valuable and are the core of all chiropractic work, you might benefit more from a holistic chiropractor who also uses other methods.

- How do you feel about the relationship between the mind and the body?
- What are some of the techniques you use?

The answers will vary, but some of the techniques that might help you with headaches are: motion palpation, Gonstead, spinal manipulation and adjustments, craniosacral therapy, myofascial release, trigger-point therapy, applied kinesiology, sacro-occipital technique, activator, body biomechanics, extremity work, and nutritional counseling. Not all chiropractors use all of these techniques, but the more treatment resources they offer, the better.

- Do you give your patients self-help procedures to do at home?
- Have you treated many chronic headache patients? What were your results?

- What are your consultations and examinations like?

You might also ask if your particular plan of insurance covers chiropractic care. Most comprehensive health plans *do* cover chiropractic treatments.

After a consultation and examination, your chiropractor will review the data and present a report of the findings, usually on your next visit. This report will inform you whether your chiropractor feels he or she can help you, what exactly is causing your headaches, the various techniques that will be used, how your headaches may be helped by this work, and approximately how long the treatment program will be. Of course, no health practitioner can guarantee success, but your chiropractor should be willing to discuss with you whether your headaches can be eliminated and how long it will take to correct the underlying causes.

A Chiropractic Case History

Isaac K. was generally a healthy young man. He ate well and took vitamin supplements, played sports regularly, and did relaxation exercises to counteract the stress he experienced in his job as a sales representative. Despite all this, he had tension headaches on a regular basis.

After a complete chiropractic examination, including x-rays, it was determined that the cause of Isaac's headaches was two pinched nerves in his neck and upper back regions, with degenerative changes in the discs between the vertebrae. The pinched nerves had developed as a result of improper biomechanics of the cervical (neck) and thoracic (upper back) regions of his spine. This led to complex alterations in the functioning of his nervous and circulatory systems, as well

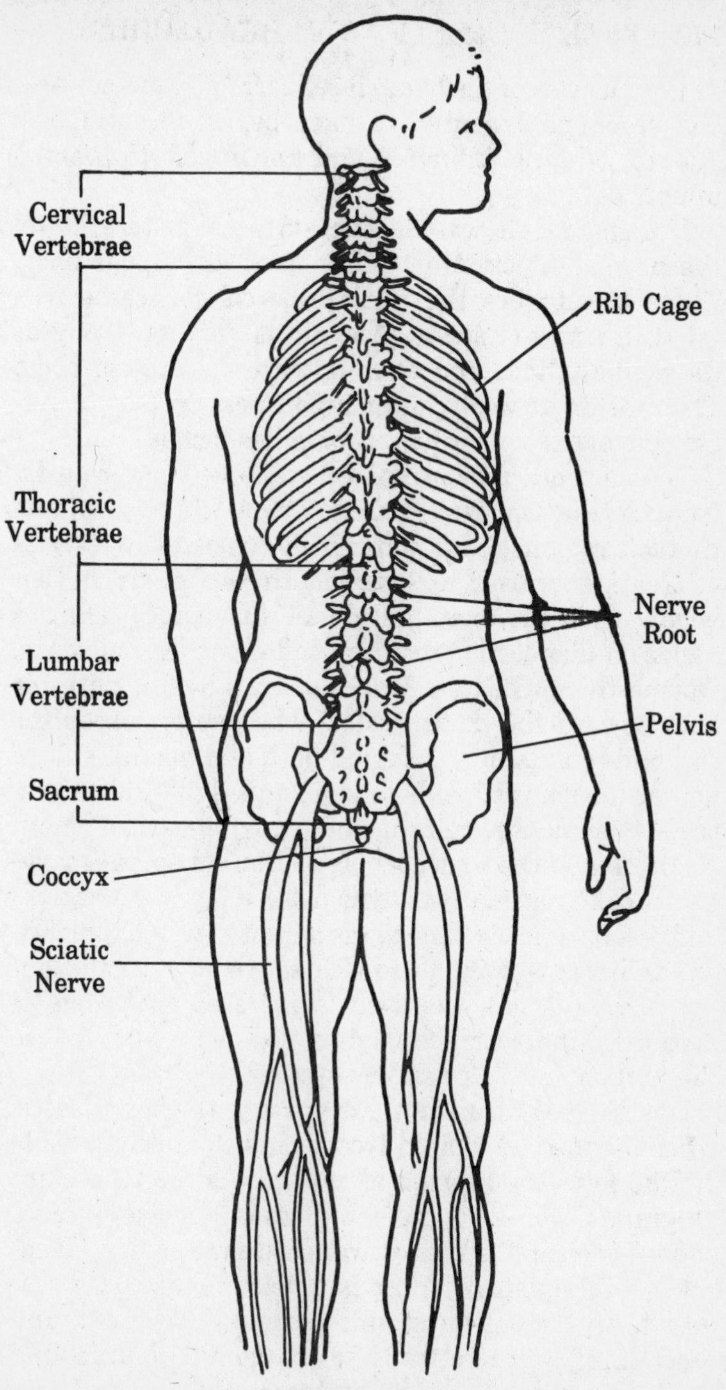
Cervical
Vertebrae
Rib Cage
Thoracic
Vertebrae
Nerve
Root
Lumbar
Vertebrae
Pelvis
Sacrum
Coccyx
Sciatic
Nerve

The Spine

as the muscles of his head, face, neck, and upper back. His problems appeared to have begun in childhood, due to athletic injuries, and continued to worsen unnoticed.

The end result was degeneration and alteration of the normal functioning of his neck and upper back. These areas were the weak links that became irritated in times of stress. A chain is only as strong as its weakest link, and so it is with the human body. The tension at work put enough stress on Isaac's vulnerable areas to produce chronic headaches.

The chiropractor designed a treatment program for Isaac to restore normal functioning to the cervical and thoracic regions of his spine. This consisted of a series of treatments over a three-month period. Each visit began with an examination of his spine, using a hands-on diagnostic procedure called motion palpation. During this procedure, Isaac sat on the table with his back toward the chiropractor, who gently placed his two hands on Issac's back and neck and had him move forward, backward, side to side, and right and left, in order to evaluate the range of motion of each segment of his spine. The exact levels of limited spinal movement (called a fixation, hypomobility, or subluxation) and resulting irritations to his nervous system (pinched and irritated nerves) were located. Gentle specific spinal manipulation was used to increase the range of motion of the restricted spinal segments and reduce the irritation to his nervous system.

Isaac looked forward to his visits to the chiropractic office because the spinal treatments were comfortable and he felt very relaxed afterward. As the treatment program progressed, he found that he was able to endure the same stress at work without getting headaches as frequently. After Isaac completed the three-month treatment program, normal movement and functioning were restored to his spinal column and the pinched nerves and resulting irritations to his nervous system were corrected. The negative effects that the spinal problem was having on his circulatory system, particularly his vertebral arteries, were corrected at the same time. Isaac was able to continue with the work and lifestyle he enjoyed with one major difference: no more headaches to disrupt his days.

Motion Palpation

Motion palpation is a diagnostic technique that was originally researched and developed by a Belgian chiropractor, Dr. Henri Gillet, and advanced by Dr. Leonard John Faye, a prominent chiropractor in Los Angeles. Motion palpation tells the practitioner which levels of the spine have normal ranges of motion and which are restricted intersegmentally. This technique enables the chiropractor to determine which level of the spine is causing irritation to the nervous system and where manipulation is needed. Thus, manipulation can be applied at the level of dysfunction. Motion palpation has allowed for great advances in the proper diagnosis of the following types of headaches:

- Cervicogenic headaches, which arise from irritation and inflammation of the nerves of the neck due to malfunction of the cervical region of the spine
- Headaches due to irritation of the nerves located in front of the cervical spine (the sympathetic ganglion chain)
- Headaches stemming from restricted movement of the first ribs located at the base of the neck, causing tight, overcontracted muscles

- Headaches caused by malfunctioning of the thoracic or upper back region of the spine
- Myalgic headaches resulting from improper functioning of the muscles

Such headaches can be migrainelike in nature and are often misdiagnosed, but chiropractors who use motion palpation and other approaches can recognize the causes of these types of headaches and treat them properly.

Craniosacral Therapy

Craniosacral therapy grew out of research performed by Dr. John Upledger, an osteopathic physician, and others at the Michigan State University Department of Biomechanics. They advanced the work of Dr. William Sutherland and developed a therapeutic modality that focuses on the normalization of the craniosacral system, as well as the network of fascia throughout the body.

According to the model developed by Dr. Upledger, the craniosacral system is a hydraulic system containing cerebrospinal fluid enclosed by the membranes that surround the brain and spinal cord. (A hydraulic system is one in which pressure exerted on a fluid-filled container causes movement in another area of the system.) The membranes of the craniosacral system are attached to bones in several places, including the bones of the skull and the sacrum (tailbone).

When there are restrictions in the membrane system or abnormalities in the functioning of the fluid-filled hydraulic system, headaches are often the result. Imbalances in the skull, pelvis, and various segments of the body structure can lead to abnormal fluid pres-

The Skull

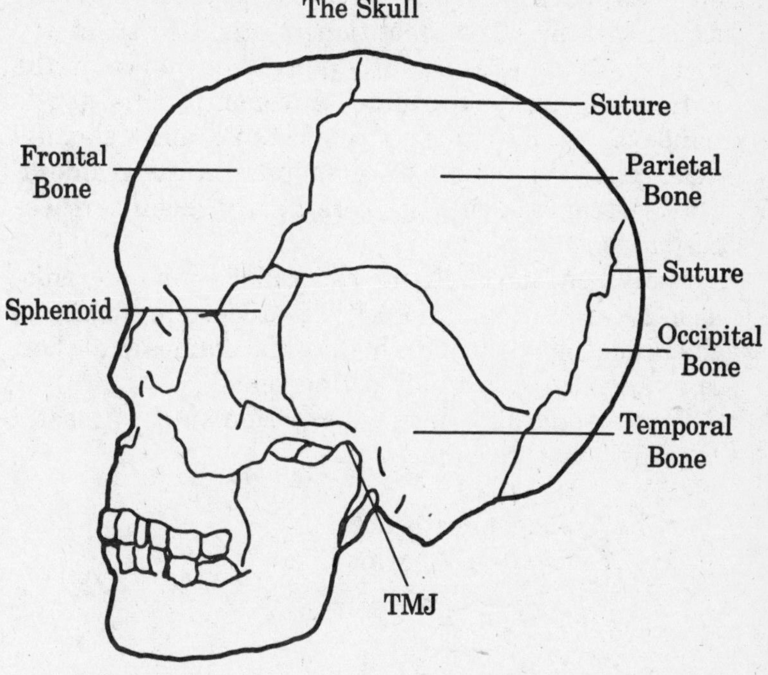

sure, membrane tension, and neurological disorganization. Such imbalances can usually be corrected by a skilled professional mobilizing any bony restrictions of the skull, pelvis, spine, and other related structures and releasing any membrane restrictions that might be present. The result of craniosacral therapy is often a positive change in the pressure buildup within the cerebrospinal fluid, which is responsible for protecting and nourishing the central nervous system. Craniosacral therapy is a noninvasive technique that is done with gentle hands-on work. "The practitioner acts as a facilitator to enhance the self-correcting activity of the system," says Dr. Upledger.

Health practitioners utilizing craniosacral therapy evaluate the cranial rhythm, movement of the cranial bones, TMJ, tension within the fascia, as well as other structures affecting the system by having patients lie on their backs, usually on a comfortable, specially designed table. The practitioners stand or sit at the head of the table and gently place their hands on the patient's head to evaluate movement. This gentle hands-on examination is comfortable and relaxing. Once problems have been diagnosed in the craniosacral system, the practitioners gently mobilize these restrictions.

Many headache patients can benefit from a craniosacral system evaluation. If the underlying cause of the headache lies within this system, craniosacral therapy can provide fast and lasting relief.

If you would like more information on craniosacral therapy, you can contact:

The Upledger Institute
11211 Prosperity Farms Road
Palm Beach Gardens, FLA 33410
(305) 622-4334

Proper dental work can play an important role in the functioning of the craniosacral system. If dental work does not result in a balanced TMJ, structural problems including imbalances in the cranium may occur, leading to headaches.

There are a small but growing number of holistic dentists who are trained in the relationship between dentistry and the proper functioning of the craniosacral system. These holistically oriented dentists often work with other practitioners to create balance in the TMJ and cranium. Holistic dentists usually avoid the use of materials such as mercury, which can cause headaches stemming from chemical imbalances and allergic responses.

Myofascial Release

Myofascial release, a new form of treatment for pain and dysfunction, focuses on the fascial system. One of its chief developers was John Barnes, P.T., a physical therapist, lecturer, and educator based in Paoli, Pennsylvania, where he founded the Myofascial Release Treatment Center.

Fascia is connective body tissue made of collagen. It surrounds and connects every muscle, organ, gland, bone, and nerve, running uninterrupted throughout the entire body. "The fascia creates scaffolding of the body, a three-dimensional web," said Mr. Barnes.

The fascia can become restricted and develop adhesions as a result of trauma (accidents and injuries), surgery, scars, inflammation, poor posture, or emotional stress. Fascial restrictions, which are very common, can create enormous pressure on pain-sensitive parts of the body and lead to symptoms anywhere in the body: back pain, neck pain, TMJ dysfunction, and headaches. Headaches can be caused by fascial restrictions in the neck, head, or other regions.

While performing myofascial release, the health professional evaluates the whole body for fascial restrictions. Then a subtle, gentle stretching technique is done with the hands to release the restrictions. "This procedure alleviates pressure and returns the body to a three-dimensional balance, which enables the self-correcting mechanisms to return to proper functioning," said Mr. Barnes. The result for headache patients, as well as other chronic pain victims, can be impressive.

Until recently, the tremendous importance of the fascial system was largely unrecognized and ignored. Now, due to the efforts of Dr. John Upledger, John Barnes, and others, many chiropractors, osteopaths, physical therapists, and other bodyworkers are using myofascial release techniques. We believe that this approach should be a part of any comprehensive treatment program for chronic headaches.

A Headache Success Story

Alice J., a stewardess, suffered from migraine headache attacks at least twice a week, and sometimes more frequently, for over two years. "When a migraine would hit in the middle of a flight I simply couldn't function. Of course, I went to the doctor, but the only thing he could do for me was give me some pills that made me feel nauseous, especially when I was flying. I simply couldn't cope and I finally had to quit my job. My husband and I thought staying home and living quietly would make me feel better. But the headaches kept coming no matter how quiet my life was," said Alice. "My sister-in-law thought her chiropractor might help me. I thought chiropractors were for backaches, so I didn't jump at the idea. But after a couple of months of staying home and going stir-crazy, I was ready to try anything."

Chiropractic examination of Alice revealed abnormal functioning of her craniosacral system. There were restrictions in the normal motion of her cranial (skull) bones, which created imbalances in her cerebrospinal fluid. The muscles of her head, jaw, neck, and upper back were overcontracted. There was restricted motion of the joint between her atlas (first vertebral bone in the neck) and her skull, which exerted an abnormal pull on her dural tube (the membrane surrounding the spinal cord). There were also myofascial adhesions and restrictions in her TMJ, neck, shoulder girdle, and the muscles of her head and face. It was evident that her migraine headaches were a result of these imbalances and restrictions.

Alice's treatment program involved craniosacral therapy, myofascial release techniques, chiropractic manipulation, TMJ work, and dural tube release. (Dural tube release is the gentle releasing and untwisting of the membranes surrounding the spinal cord.) Alice's migraine attacks tapered off and, after several months of treatment, ceased altogether.

"I think a lot of people suffer unnecessarily because they think nothing can get rid of migraines or because they're afraid to try anything new. But there's really nothing to be afraid of. None of the treatments I received were at all painful or even uncomfortable. And there were no side effects to worry about. Best of all, the treatments worked," said Alice. "I was able to go back to work and start feeling good about my life again. Now when I smile at a passenger, I really mean it!"

Trying New Techniques

Many people are reluctant to try new professional treatments for their headaches. This may be due to a fear of the unknown and/or the belief that nothing can cure headaches. We hope that, like Alice, you can overcome these negative thoughts and reap the rewards of alternative headache treatments.

Because the holistic health care field is so large today, it can be confusing to look for professional help without guidance. To make this search simpler and easier for you, we have developed a complimentary referral system that lists chiropractors, osteopaths, physical therapists, and other holistic health professionals in different areas of the country.

If you would like more information, you can call or write to:

Dr. Jan Stromfeld
330 West 58th Street
Suite 4G
New York, NY 10019
(212) 765-6470

Chapter Eleven

If Your Children Have Headaches

HEADACHES TEND TO BE ASSOCIATED WITH THE PRESSURE and tension of adult life. But the sad reality is that many children also endure chronic headaches. According to the National Center for Health, children lost approximately 1.3 million days of school in 1986 because of headaches.

In contrast to the adult ratio, the ratio of male to female migraineurs in childhood is almost even, with a slight preponderance of males. Around puberty this changes, and in adulthood about three times as many women as men have migraines. This may be due to hormonal fluctuations resulting from imbalances within women's endocrine systems.

Children can suffer from almost any type of headache, but the majority of cases, and perhaps the most frightening, involve migraines. Approximately one-fourth of all adult migraineurs started having attacks when they were children. Migraine attacks can begin as early as twelve months, although the average age of the first attack is about six years.

Children's migraines share most of the characteristics of adults', although they are generally shorter in duration. This is little consolation, however, since to children, an hour of agony may seem like forever. Nausea, vomiting, and extreme sensitivity to light usually accompany childhood migraines. In some cases there are temporary speech difficulties, partial paralysis, and disruptions in vision and the other senses.

Vertebrobasilar migraine is a particularly traumatic form of migraine that often besets youngsters. In addition to head pain, vertebrobasilar migraines can cause neurological symptoms such as vertigo, loss of balance and coordination, temporary paralysis, speech difficulties, and even unconsciousness. This type of migraine can be the result of hypomobility (decreased motion) of the joint between the first bone of the neck (atlas) and the base of the skull (occiput). This can potentially cause irritation to the brain stem, spinal cord, and craniosacral rhythm. This condition can often be corrected by conservative chiropractic treatment.

Why the Holistic Approach Is Right for Children

If you are like most parents, you would do almost anything to make your children feel better when they hurt. You are probably tempted to take the easy way out and give your children painkillers when they have headaches. Although this is an understandable reaction, in the long run it may not be the healthiest way of dealing with your children's pain. If children begin to think that drugs are the answer to pain, suffering, and problems, they may be more likely to abuse drugs in later years. In addition to the psychological side effects of giving your children painkillers, there are the physical ones to consider. Children are especially sensitive to the various side effects of headache medications that were outlined earlier. Why take chances with your children's health? Why not explore safe, natural alternatives instead?

By choosing holistic approaches, you will teach your

children many valuable lessons, in addition to helping their headaches. They will receive the message that pain can often be eliminated and prevented without drugs and learn to take an active role in maintaining their health. By getting in touch with their feelings, they can become aware how their emotions affect their health. They will make discoveries about how their bodies work and how good nutrition and other healthy habits can make them feel better.

Your children can carry these lessons with them throughout their lives and use them to solve and avoid many problems. By taking the time to help your children with their headaches in a holistic manner, you may profoundly enhance the quality of their entire lives.

Professional Help for Your Children

If your children have headaches, the first step is to take them to a medical doctor for a complete checkup, to rule out the possibility of any serious illness. This will put both you and your children at ease.

It is also important to be sure your children are examined by a qualified optometrist or ophthalmologist to be certain that eyestrain is not the cause of their headaches. Children's eyes change much more rapidly than adults' eyes do and often need vision correction. Be aware that because children are sometimes reluctant to wear glasses, they may not tell you that they're not seeing well.

After the checkups by medical and eye doctors, we recommend that you take your children to a holistic chiropractor to see if they have any structural problems. No matter how young children are, they may have subluxations, imbalances, or cranial problems that contribute to headaches. Problems can begin as early as the birth process. When the obstetrician pulls the baby by the head and neck during delivery, pinched nerves and cranial imbalances that can cause headaches later in life often develop. Children are also prone to structural problems due to the active nature of their lives. Rough horseplay and sports are natural activities for children, but they can create problems that remain undetected until you visit a professional.

Posture, Exercise, and Massage

Once your children have been helped by a chiropractor, you'll want to help them maintain balanced and relaxed bodies. One way you can do this is to encourage good posture. Postural habits are established in childhood, and this is the optimal time to correct them.

When you check your children's posture from the side view, notice:

- Do their lower backs and buttocks sway out, or are they tucked under?
- Are their heads jutting forward or are their necks lifted and aligned?
- Do their shoulders round forward, or are they straight?
- Do their chests thrust out too far or cave in, or are they straight?
- Are their knees hyperextended (locked backward), or are they relaxed and slightly bent?

When you check them from the front, look for these clues:

- Is one shoulder higher than the other, or are their shoulders even?
- Do their chests look sunken, or lifted?
- Do their abdomens appear to be hanging forward, or do they look firm?
- Are they slouching onto one hip, or standing upright?
- Is the weight of their body centered over their ankle joints, or do they rest too far back on their heels?

You will also want to check your children's posture when they do their homework, read, eat, and watch television. Are any of their positions putting a strain on their necks? How do they sleep? Sleeping on their sides or back is okay, but sleeping on their stomachs can cause neck strain and headaches.

When you correct your children's posture, try to be very gentle. Give them time; don't expect them to change all at once. If they are old enough to understand, explain the connection between bad posture and headaches so they know why you are concerned. You might also add that bad posture can cause back pain and overall weakness.

Instead of making postural change a harsh, punitive experience, try to make it a pleasant one. Give them positive reinforcement by making comments such as: "You look so tall and handsome when you lift your head up," or "You look so graceful and pretty, like a dancer, when you tuck in your lower back." Gentle and loving messages often have the most impact.

Exercise and Children's Headaches

Children are usually more active than adults, but their exercise is not usually the type that helps headaches. The competitive and rough nature of their physical activities may actually add to their headache problems. Gentle stretching helps counteract the abuse your children's bodies take during their play. You might teach them the exercise routine presented in Chapter Nine, which is appropriate for children as well as adults.

Don't try to force your children into stretching; they may come to think of it as a chore, something to be avoided. Instead, present stretching as a fun and joyful game. If your children continue to resist learning the stretching routine, you might pique their interest by doing it yourself and telling them how good it feels. They may want to get in on the fun. At the very least, doing the routine will make you feel better.

Massage for Your Children

One of the most loving things you can do for your children when they have headaches is to massage them. You can use the classical massage or the pressure-point sequences in Chapter Nine, or you can improvise. We recommend that you don't restrict massages to times when your children are in pain, however, since this can subconsciously encourage headaches. Instead, massages can become a wonderful way to give your children a special treat even when they are feeling fine. If they are old enough, you can teach them to return the favor. Exchanging massages is a delightful way for your family to express mutual love while promoting good health.

It's also a good idea to teach your children self-massage. Children often have highly developed motor skills at a young age and are quick learners. Present self-massage as a special game, one where everyone wins.

Psychological Elements

Peter E. first started getting migraine headaches when his family moved to a new town. He was seven years old and had to start the second grade with a group of children who already knew each other. As the new boy in school, he was made the class scapegoat; school was a nightmare. As a result of the emotional stress, he developed structural and chemical imbalances leading to migraine headaches.

His mother had suffered from migraines all her life and was very sympathetic. She allowed Peter to stay home from school whenever his head hurt. Instead of the ostracism of his classmates, he could spend the day luxuriating in the loving attention of his mother. It was almost worth the pain.

Gradually, Peter became accepted by his classmates. His headaches became infrequent and he rarely missed school. But when he was eleven, his parents' marriage became strained and they began to fight a great deal. Peter started getting severe headaches again as a result of his body's reaction to stress.

Children's headaches, like adults', are often linked to their emotional lives. This does not mean that their headaches are not real or that the children are "faking it." The pain is real and so are the physical changes, although they may be caused by psychological stress.

Headaches can be a way for children to avoid doing something they are afraid to do, such as facing the pressures of school or dealing with difficult peers. Children may use headaches as a means to avoid responsibilities such as homework, chores, or afterschool jobs. Headaches may serve the purpose of giving children an escape route from social situations that make them uncomfortable. When children feel they are not getting enough love or affection, they may use headaches to gain more. If children feel that their parents are preoccupied with their own problems and lives, headaches may be a desperate cry for attention. It should be understood that these headaches are usually due to physiological changes in the body that take place because of stressful situations and psychological problems.

The best way to determine if there are psychological reasons behind your children's headaches is to talk to them. Try to approach these discussions in a relaxed manner. If your children are very reluctant to talk, encourage them by saying that you love them no matter what they say, feel, or do. If they absolutely refuse to talk, wait and try another time.

If your children are of school age, ask them questions such as: How was school this week? Do you have too much homework? Are you worried about any tests? Is your teacher nice? Judging by their responses, you can decide if it is necessary for you to speak to their teachers or counselors.

If your children express anxieties about school, try to reassure them that you love them no matter how well they do academically. Tell them that your love is absolute and unwavering and does not depend on grades or other achievements. Knowing that they do not have to "earn" your love will greatly reduce their anxiety. Such reassurance can help prevent your children from becoming perfectionists who set unrealistic goals for themselves and others and then become tense when these goals are not realized. It can give them a core of security that helps eliminate the anxiety that can exacerbate headaches and other stress-related disorders.

Question your children about their peer relationships to see if they are making them emotionally upset. Ask them if they like their classmates; if anyone is giving them a hard time; if they are getting along with their friends; if they have enough friends; if they feel lonely.

Although you should not directly interfere with your children's peer relationships, simply talking can be very therapeutic. A regular parent-child dialogue can establish a healthy pattern of talking about relationships instead of keeping feelings bottled up inside. You can teach your children that they should feel free to discuss anything, whether it is happy or sad. This can prevent them from holding anger, fear, and anxiety inside, where it can create ill health.

You should also communicate with your children about their feelings about you and the rest of the family. You can ask them questions such as: Do you miss us when we go to work? Do you feel we're spending enough time with you? Do you know that we love each other very much? Do you know we love you very much? How are you getting along with your brothers and sisters?

These questions may bring up some disturbing responses for which there are no easy answers. But again, answers are not always necessary. Expressing feelings in itself can be extremely beneficial—especially if you respond to your children's comments with reassurances of love, hugs, and kisses.

When their children are in pain, some parents say, "Let me kiss it and make it all better." Then they kiss the spot that hurts. This is a classic expression of the healing power of love and affection, and it can certainly be a wonderful remedy. However, if children only receive enough affection when they are sick or hurt, they may become ill more frequently in an unconscious attempt to receive this nurturing love. You need to be appropriately sympathetic without smothering them with love, or they may learn to enjoy being sick. Or they may come to associate pain with love, with negative repercussions on their later relationships, as well as their health. One of the healthiest things you can do for your children is to give them verbal expressions of love and physical affection as often as possible, not only when they are sick or hurt.

When Headaches Run in the Family

Perhaps one of the most difficult times to be loving to your children is when you have a headache yourself. We hope this book will help you alleviate your own pain and put you in a stronger position to take care of your children. If or when you do have severe headaches, however, it is best to tell them the truth and explain why you are not feeling well. If you don't tell them that you have a headache, they might imagine you have an even more serious ailment, or they may think you are angry at them because they did something wrong. It is usually best to tell them the truth, without dwelling too much on the pain you are experiencing. Try not to give the headache too much importance or power in their minds. This may be difficult, especially if you have a migraine, but no one ever said being a parent was easy.

The most important point is to avoid instilling in your children the belief that because you suffer from headaches, they will, too. It is estimated that about half of all children who suffer from chronic headaches have a family history of this problem, and there may well be a genetic component. But there is no reason that young children should be saddled with this depressing news when you can encourage them to believe that they can live healthy, pain-free lives.

Sugar and Children's Headaches

Melissa T. was the pampered baby of her family, an adorable little blonde girl. Because she was rather skinny, her parents allowed her to have extra helpings of dessert and candy. Melissa often felt tired and had frequent headaches. Ironically, her mother also gave her extra chocolate candy bars as a consolation whenever her head hurt.

Her concerned third-grade teacher noticed that Melissa was absent frequently. She also noticed that Melissa always had a candy bar, another sweet such as cupcakes or cookies, and sugary soda at lunchtime. The teacher suggested to Melissa's mother that this diet might be contributing to the child's health problems.

"I was very surprised when the teacher said she thought too much sugar might be giving Melissa headaches. So I took her to my doctor and he did some tests. He found out she was hypoglycemic. That explained why she felt weak and tired a lot, as well as the headaches," said Melissa's mother.

"I tried to explain to Melissa that sweets were making her head hurt and making her feel tired. This was hard for her to take and she had a fit when I said she shouldn't eat sweets. So I bribed her. I promised her I would take her to Disneyland if she would stop eating them. So she did. And she stopped getting the headaches and felt a lot perkier. Of course, after the Disneyland trip she wanted to start eating sweets again and I couldn't stop her. But when she did, she'd get headaches and feel awful. Well, she's a bright little girl and eventually she decided that the sweets really did make her feel sick, so she didn't want to eat them anymore."

Children, like adults, are often allergic to the very

things that they crave most, such as sugar. Sugar frequently causes hypoglycemia and food allergy symptoms. If your children have headaches, you should try to eliminate sugar from their lives as much as possible. This may not be an easy task, but you can try. Offer them fresh fruits for dessert and snacks. If there are sugary foods in your house, it will be very hard for your children to resist them, so try to keep these out of your cupboards. Of course, once your children are out of the house they may succumb to temptation. If they do, try not to be too harsh; just explain that sugar is bad for them and may cause them to have headaches.

Food Allergies and Children's Headaches

Children can be highly sensitive to many types of food. Sometimes these food allergies are linked to an overgrowth of candida albicans in the children's digestive systems, often due to the overuse of antibiotics. It is now widely recognized that food allergies can cause many of the characteristics associated with "difficult" children, such as hyperactivity, short attention span, irritability, hostility, and anxiety. Food allergies can also cause physical symptoms such as respiratory problems, digestive disorders, muscle pains, and headaches in children.

If your children have headaches, we recommend that you see a qualified nutritionist to have them tested for food allergies, as many allergists readily acknowledge that nutritionists are more familiar with food allergies. Children can undergo the same elimination diet that we recommend for adults in Chapter Six, but this may not be practical because this diet demands a degree of commitment and self-control that is unrealistic to expect of most youngsters.

Once your nutritionist determines what substances your children are allergic to, you can take steps to eliminate these from their diets. If your children are very young you can simply stop feeding them these substances. If they are older, it is more complicated. First, you should explain that these foods or drinks can cause them to have headaches and that is why they shouldn't have them anymore. Tell them that you are not taking away these items as a punishment, but in order to make them feel better. If possible, try not to serve these foods or drinks to the rest of the family. Try to keep them out of the house altogether. When your children eat out, encourage them to avoid problem foods by making clear the connection between these allergic substances and headaches.

Your nutritionist will probably recommend vitamin and mineral supplementation for your children. Deficiencies of these vital elements are very common and can cause headaches. Supplementary needs vary according to your children's ages and specific requirements.

One of the best things you can do for your children's headaches and their overall health (and yours, as well) is to set an example of healthy eating. Follow the guidelines in Chapter Six, or further explore good nutrition in other books. Raise your children on natural, fresh foods without extra sugar, salt, preservatives, or additives. It is true that they will probably experiment with junk foods once they reach a certain age. But if they were raised on healthy food, once they are past this rebellious stage they will probably return to a healthy diet. In any case, their physiological makeup will have a strong, healthy foundation.

Environment and Children's Headaches

Like adults, children can be allergic to substances in their environment, as well as their food and drink. Inhaled particles such as dust, mold, pollen, fur, and feathers can trigger allergic reactions. Chemical pollutants and toxic minerals can also be allergens. Allergies to these environmental substances can cause health disorders such as headaches, as well as emotional problems.

Unfortunately, in today's overindustrialized and polluted world it is nearly impossible to avoid all possible allergens. You can take steps to reduce your children's exposure, however. This may help you clear up other health problems in addition to headaches.

Here are some suggestions:

- Buy an electrostatic air cleaner for your children's bedroom and any other room they frequently use.
- Clean your house regularly to reduce dust, animal danders, and other allergens. Don't forget to clean air conditioners, humidifiers, dehumidifiers, radiators, and heating vents.
- Avoid molds by keeping the bathroom and basement as dry, clean, and well-ventilated as possible.
- Consider switching to unscented, natural cleaning agents, which you can find in many health food stores. In these stores you can also find natural soaps, shampoos, and deodorants to replace chemical-laden products.
- If possible, give your children 100 percent cotton bedding and all-cotton clothing instead of synthetics.

- In extreme cases, allergy-related headaches can be caused by rugs, carpets, heavy draperies, stuffed furniture, animal hairs, plastic dishes and utensils, as well as aluminum foil and cookware. If necessary, use stainless steel, ceramic, glass, and wooden dishes and cookware, and cellophane wraps instead.
- Consider installing water filters on your faucets and/or use natural spring water.
- If your children come home from school with headaches, look into the possibility that they are being exposed to chemicals in art, shop, or science classes. See if their classrooms are well ventilated and well lit. Check into the possibility of cleaning agents, copying materials, or computers bothering your children. If changes need to be made, approach the school personnel in a friendly noncombative manner and express appreciation for their support. Your efforts may help other children as well as your own.

Try not to be overwhelmed by the task of cleaning up your children's environment and diet; make changes at a pace that is comfortable and practical for you. The main guideline is that their world, from their meals to their clothing to their bedrooms, should be as natural and free of chemical pollutants as possible.

Chapter Twelve

The Holistic Headache Recovery Program

The Holistic Headache Recovery Program offers a step-by-step plan to help you live a headache-free life. The program is only a guide; you can adapt it any way you choose. No timetable is given for the recovery steps; do not feel any pressure to make more changes than you can handle at any given time. Develop your own personal timetable and proceed with the program at a pace that is comfortable and practical for you.

The steps of the Holistic Headache Recovery Program are designed to build on each other and work together. Rather than abandoning one step when you move on to the next one, you should keep adding to your repertoire of self-help measures.

The only prerequisite for the recovery program is a positive attitude. Affirmations and creative imagery can help plant positive thoughts in your subconscious and keep negativity from sabotaging your efforts. Use the tremendous power of your mind to assist you in eliminating headaches from your life forever.

Step One: Enlist Professional Help

Before you begin self-help practices or seek alternative treatments, you should have a thorough checkup from a medical doctor to ascertain if your headaches are symptomatic of any serious illness. You may want to go to your trusted family M.D. for this checkup. But if you don't already have a physician with whom you are satisfied, this may be a good time to establish a relationship with a holistic medical doctor.

According to the American Holistic Medical Association, an estimated ten thousand, or 2 percent, of doctors in the United States can be considered holistic. This number is increasing rapidly as evidence of the value of holistic modalities accumulates. In 1987, the National Institutes of Health spent over $70 million researching "behavioral medicine," including biofeedback, relaxation training, and hypnosis. This is a welcome indication that the medical establishment is beginning to pay more attention to the connection between the mind and body.

The American Holistic Medical Association and Foundation offers referrals to holistic physicians across the country. For more information, you can call or write to:

American Holistic Medical Association and Foundation
2002 Eastlake Avenue E
Seattle, WA 98102
(206) 322-6842

If you are looking for a new medical doctor but are unable to find a holistic physician in your area, you can look for a practitioner who is at least open to the holistic approach, someone who will not discourage you from including holistic alternatives in your health care regime. Don't be shy about asking questions; you have every right to be an informed health care consumer.

You might ask, "What do you think of holistic health

care?" If the response is something like, "It's a bunch of hogwash," this may not be an appropriate doctor for you. If the answer is along the lines of "I don't know much about it," you might look for a better-informed doctor who keeps in touch with a wider array of information.

Another question you might ask is, "Do you believe that emotions play an important role in health? What about nutrition and exercise?" While most doctors will readily admit that these are vital considerations, their responses will help you decide how knowledgeable they are about these subjects.

"What are your feelings about prescribing drugs for headaches?" is another question that may elicit a telling response. Answers such as, "Fine, I do it all the time," or "A prescription's the easiest way to help someone," show a certain lack of respect for natural healing. A more enlightened response might be, "I only prescribe painkillers when absolutely necessary."

Next, you may want to ask, "How would you feel if I also went to a chiropractor, nutritionist, or massage therapist?" You need to be sure that the medical doctor you choose does not discourage you from enjoying the benefits of other valuable approaches. You might also ask doctors if they refer their patients to holistic practitioners.

After your medical doctor rules out the possibility that any serious illness is the cause of your headaches, we recommend that you visit a holistic chiropractor. Your chiropractor can help correct structural imbalances that may be contributing to your headaches. Your chiropractor can also determine if you need to enlist other professionals, such as a massage therapist, a nutritionist, or a holistic dentist, in your fight against headaches.

Step Two: Take Stock of Your Mental Attitude

The onset of the recovery program is a good time to take stock of how you view yourself, others, and the world in general. One way to do this is to explore your inner feelings in a personal journal. Since this journal will be for your eyes only, there is no need to censor yourself or worry about grammar or style. If you simply let the words flow, you may discover feelings and emotions that were previously blocked or repressed. If you really dislike writing, you can set aside a time period to have an inner dialogue with yourself about psychological issues.

You can use the following questions as starting points or catalysts for this psychological exploration:

- Are you a perfectionist? Are you often judgmental or overdemanding with yourself or others? Are you often disappointed in yourself or others?
- Do you cling to rigid thinking or unhappy situations because of fear or insecurity? Are you often anxious or afraid? Do you think of the world as a hostile place?
- Do you have low self-esteem? Do you love yourself enough? Are you good to yourself?
- Do you receive enough love and respect from other people? Are your relationships satisfying? Do you express your needs fully and honestly to the people in your life?
- Do you usually start the day with a feeling of dread? Are you harboring a great deal of anger, fear, or anxiety? Are you often depressed?

Answering these questions honestly will help you determine whether unresolved emotional issues are undermining your health. Self-discovery takes a great deal of courage and commitment. Be gentle and kind with yourself during this process, and use relaxation, creative imagery, and affirmation techniques to strengthen your inner resources.

You may discover disturbing thoughts and feelings that you have long been trying to repress. If this is the case, don't be afraid to reach out for help. Professional counseling and peer support groups can provide support and guidance. Psychological self-help books are available to assist with almost any problem. Talking to your friends and family can also be very comforting.

It is not necessary for you to solve every psychological issue in order to stop getting headaches. The point is to open up and get in touch with your feelings, so that they don't have to send you a message of pain in order to be noticed.

Step Three: Begin Practicing Relaxation Exercises

Step Two may initially increase your anxiety level, so it is important that you start doing relaxation exercises to counteract the stress.

Begin by practicing deep breathing, since this facilitates all other relaxation techniques. Then choose the relaxation method from Chapter Seven that appeals to you most and try to practice it once a day. Give it a week or so, and if you find that it still doesn't "work" for you, try another technique. Remember not to try to force the relaxation; just let yourself float into it. If you have trouble shutting off the usual litany of thoughts and concentrating, don't become angry with yourself. Simply keep trying; relaxation will come.

Even if you experience benefits from the first form

of relaxation you try, you might experiment with other techniques and find that you reach even deeper levels of inner peace.

Try to do a relaxation technique at least once a day, and twice a day whenever possible. If you're undergoing a very stressful time, perhaps you can treat yourself to slightly longer periods of relaxation. Even when you are busy, try to make time to give yourself a twenty-minute relaxation break each day. Remember that relaxation can strengthen your inner resources and make it easier to cope with all the other demands of your lifestyle.

Step Four: Begin Doing Affirmations and Creative Imagery

If you have not started doing so at the onset of the recovery program, we recommend that you begin doing affirmations and creative imagery at this point. These practices have two major functions: They enable your subconscious mind to help you beat headaches, and they help you improve areas of your life that may be contributing to your stress and pain.

If you found that the creative imagery and affirmation techniques in Chapter Seven go strongly against your grain, you have, of course, the choice not to do them. Perhaps a method such as neuro-linguistic programming, which may seem more scientific, suits your style better. If you go to any bookstore, you will see that there are books on scores of different mind techniques.

Step Five: Make Necessary Changes in Your Diet

It is easier to undergo this difficult but vital step with the guidance of a holistic professional. If your doctor does not do nutritional counseling, you might ask for a referral to a qualified nutritionist. But if you choose to "do it yourself," refer to Chapter Six for the specifics.

Here are the general components of this step:

- Eliminate the foods that are commonly known to be migraine triggers from your diet.
- Eliminate potentially toxic substances from your diet.
- Track down your food allergies with the Food Elimination Diet or professional help. A health professional can also determine if you have a candida albicans problem and/or if you are hypoglycemic. Stop consuming the substances to which you are allergic. If you have a candida problem or are hypoglycemic, make the necessary dietary changes to correct these conditions.
- Develop a healthy, balanced, natural diet for yourself. Drink about a quart of fresh spring water daily.
- Take proper vitamin and mineral supplementation to guard against deficiencies.

Don't try to make all these changes at the same time unless you are a highly disciplined person; otherwise, you might rebel and give up completely. Proceed at a pace where discernible progress is made, but not so quickly that you are upset.

Most likely, you will occasionally undergo setbacks and succumb to foods or drinks that you know may trigger headaches. Even if you don't experience an immediate headache as a result, don't take this as an indication that it is okay to continue consuming that substance. Sometimes the effects can be cumulative or delayed, and the reactive headache may hit later. Forgive yourself for the temporary lack of self-control, but reaffirm your commitment to preventing headaches through dietary changes.

You can use affirmations and creative imagery to bolster your willpower during this step. Or you can use a type of negative behavioral programming: Every time you crave a food that is bad for you, spend a few minutes thinking about your last headache attack. You will probably decide that a few minutes of pleasure is not worth hours of agony. You can program yourself positively by thinking about the rewards of sticking to your dietary changes. Besides reducing headaches, you might solve other health problems and end up looking and feeling tremendously better.

Step Six: Examine Your Environment

This step involves detecting if any aspects of your environment are contributing to your headaches and taking action to reduce the effects of these factors.

Begin by looking at your home. If you or anyone in your family smokes or if you live in a heavily polluted area, the air itself might be giving you headaches. There is little you can do about outside air pollution unless you want to become active in environmental groups. But you can improve the quality of the air inside your home by using electronic air-filter machines and air ionizers.

To reduce possible allergens, try to keep your home

as clean and mold-free as possible. Don't sabotage your efforts by using chemical cleaners, which might also cause allergic responses; use natural-ingredient cleansers. You might also look at the personal hygiene products and cosmetics you use to see if any of them are causing allergic reactions.

Examine the lighting in your home, particularly in areas where you read or work, to ensure it is sufficient. See if your television is situated at a proper distance from where you sit to watch it, so that eyestrain does not occur.

You will also want to examine your work environment carefully, especially if you develop headaches on the job, as many people do. Are you being exposed to any toxic chemicals on the job? Is your workplace well ventilated and smoke-free? If not, an air-filter machine might help, and so might an open window. Is your desk chair supportive and comfortable? If it is not, ask your employer for a new chair, or purchase one yourself if necessary.

If you sit in front of a video display terminal for long periods of time, check to see if it is elevated at the proper level so that you don't have to bend your neck up or down to look at it. You might also consider getting a screen that reduces glare from the VDT.

Step Seven: Develop Healthy Habits

One of the fundamentals of headache prevention is to develop healthy postural habits, since poor posture can cause bodily imbalances, strain, and pain. Check your posture according to the criteria in Chapter Eight and try to make any appropriate corrections. Don't expect to change your posture overnight, but keep gently adjusting yourself. After a time, good posture will come naturally.

Seated posture is also an important factor in headache prevention. Sit in a manner that does not put strain on your back or your neck. Keep your neck long and lifted whether you're reading, eating, playing, or talking on the phone—whatever you do. Try to be careful that you don't strain your body when you do heavy lifting. Keep your handbag or briefcase as light as possible. When you need to carry a great deal, divide it into two even loads.

Even relaxing in bed can cause neck strain and headaches if you jam too many pillows behind your head. Also, try not to sleep on your stomach, a position that puts a great deal of pressure on your neck because your head is turned to one side for many hours. If you experience neck pain or stiffness along with headaches upon waking, a cervical pillow might help.

Step Eight: Include Stretching in Your Daily Routine

Stiffness in your upper body can often lead to headaches, so try to make a practice of doing the stretching routine in Chapter Eight every day, or as often as you can. This stretching routine is hardly a boot camp workout; it is gentle, easy, and fun to do. Try to think of it as a pleasure rather than a chore. If you can, take mini-stretching breaks throughout the day whenever you feel tension building up. You might want to begin practicing yoga if you find you enjoy stretching.

Aerobic exercise can enhance your overall body functioning, as long as you don't bring a competitive, tense frame to mind to the workout. Stay in touch with your body and don't overdo it. Swimming, or even dancing around your room, can be fun and safe ways to get your endorphins flowing.

Step Nine: Begin to Experience the Benefits of Massage

By the time you reach this step, you've probably worked hard to rid yourself of headaches. You've made certain adjustments in your lifestyle that might have been difficult and you certainly deserve a treat. But instead of going on a drinking or ice cream eating binge and suffering the consequences, you will want a reward that enhances your health. Massage is the "icing on the cake," but without the calories or sugar-induced headaches.

If you are able to afford the luxury of a professional massage session, wonderful. In any case, you can try to set up a mutual massage system with a "massage buddy," as outlined in Chapter Nine.

Self-massage is a pleasure you can enjoy every day without spending money or relying on anyone else. Massage can greatly reduce head, neck, and shoulder problems and the headaches that may result, as well as provide immediate pain relief. You can give yourself massages upon waking, after coming home from work, before going to sleep, or any time you wish. You can also treat yourself to mini-massages throughout the day for soothing relaxation.

Enjoying a Pain-Free Life

Preventive health care is an ongoing process. We hope you will continue the activities of the program even after your headache problem is under control. If you adopt a healthy way of life permanently, your chances of suffering from headaches and other ailments will be greatly reduced.

Regular visits to holistic health professionals can prevent the development of structural imbalances that cause headaches and other pains. Taking care of your psychological needs and regularly doing relaxation techniques can reduce stress-related headaches and other maladies. Practicing affirmations and creative imagery can give you confidence in your control over your health as well as other aspects of your life. Good nutrition and the avoidance of allergens and toxins can clear up and prevent many other health problems in addition to headaches. Cleaning up your environment can prevent serious diseases as well as headaches from occurring. Healthy habits, good posture, and exercise can make you feel and look better all over. Massage is not only good for pain relief and prevention; it is also a pleasure.

By taking a holistic approach to preventing headaches, you can experience an infinite number of other benefits. Your mind and body can achieve a state of optimal well-being. You can enjoy a more aware, energetic, and satisfying life, with no more headaches.

Suggested Further Reading

Allergies

Crook, William G. *Solving the Puzzle of Your Hard-to-Raise Child.* New York: Random House, 1987.

———. *The Yeast Connection.* Jackson, TN: Professional Books, 1983.

Null, Gary, and Feldman, Martin. *Good Food, Good Mood.* New York: Dodd, Mead, 1988.

Randolph, Theron G., and Moss, Ralph W. *An Alternative Approach to Allergies.* New York: Bantam Books, 1987.

Craniosacral Therapy

Upledger, John E., and Vredevoogd, Jon D. *Craniosacral Therapy.* Seattle: Eastlake Press, 1983.

Upledger, John E., *Craniosacral Therapy II: Beyond the Dura.* Seattle: Eastlake Press, 1987.

Creative Imagery and Affirmations

Gawain, Shakti. *Creative Visualization.* New York: Bantam, 1982.

———. *Living in the Light.* Mill Valley, CA: Whatever Publishing, 1986.

General

Bliss, Shepherd, ed. *The New Holistic Health Handbook.* New York: Viking Penguin, 1985.

Padeus, Emrika, and Editors of *Prevention. The Complete Guide to Your Emotions and Your Health.* Emmaus, PA: Rodale Press, 1987.

Massage

Bahr, Robert. *Good Hands.* New York: New American Library, 1984.

Downing, George. *The Massage Book.* New York: Random House, 1972.

Inkeles, Gordon. *The New Massage.* New York: G. P. Putnam's Sons, 1980.

Kunz, Barbara, and Kunz, Kevin. *The Practitioner's Guide to Reflexology.* Englewood Cliffs, NJ: Prentice-Hall, 1985.

Prudden, Bonnie. *Pain Erasure.* New York: Ballantine Books, 1980.

Meditation

Ballantine, Rudolph M., ed. *Theory and Practice of Meditation.* Honesdale, PA: Himalayan Institute, 1987.

LeShan, Lawrence. *How to Meditate.* New York: Bantam, 1986.

Neuro-Linguistic Programming

Roberts, Anthony. *Unlimited Power.* New York: Ballantine Books, 1986.

Nutrition

Airola, Paavo. *Hypoglycemia: A Better Approach.* Phoenix, AZ: Health Plus, 1977.

Colbin, Annemarie. *Food and Healing.* New York: Ballantine Books, 1987.

Mindell, Earl. *The Vitamin Bible.* New York: Warner Books, 1985.

Null, Gary. *The Complete Guide to Health and Nutrition.* New York: Dell, 1984.

Self-Healing

Borysenko, Joan. *Minding the Body, Mending the Mind.* Reading, MA: Addison-Wesley, 1987.

Breslar, David E., and Trubo, Richard. *Free Yourself from Pain.* New York: Simon & Schuster, 1979.

Hay, Louise. *You Can Heal Your Life.* Santa Monica, CA: Hay House, 1984.

Siegel, Bernie S. *Love, Medicine & Miracles.* New York: Harper & Row, 1987.

Stress Reduction

Benson, Herbert. *Beyond the Relaxation Response.* New York: Berkley, 1985.

———. *The Relaxation Response.* New York: Avon, 1976.

Selye, Hans. *The Stress of Life.* New York: McGraw-Hill, 1976 (revised).

———. *Stress Without Distress.* Philadelphia: J. B. Lippincott, 1974.

Yoga and Exercise

Anderson, Bob. *Stretching.* Bolinas, CA: Shelter Publishing, 1980.

Hittleman, Richard. *Yoga for Health*. New York: Ballantine Books, 1983.

Iyengar, B.K.S. *Light of Pranayama—The Yogic Art of Breathing*. New York: Crossroads, 1988.

———. *Light on Yoga*. New York: Schocken Books, 1979.

Lidell, Lucy. *Sivananda Companion to Yoga*. New York: Simon & Schuster, 1983.

Periodicals

East West. Brookline, MA: Kushi Foundation, Inc.

New Age. Brighton, MA: Rising Star, Inc.

Prevention. Emmaus, PA: Rodale Press.

Total Health: Mind, Body Spirit. Woodland Hills, CA: Trio Publications.

Yoga Journal. Berkeley, CA: California Yoga Teachers Association.

Index